Bird's Eye View of
Rheumatology

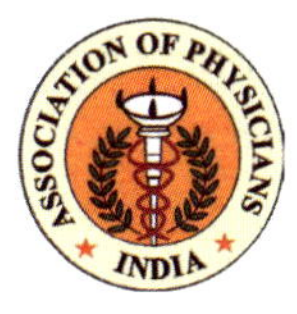

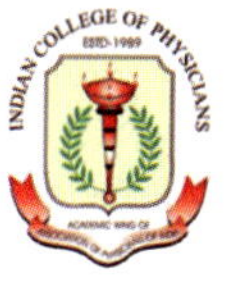

Foreword

Rheumatology, a dynamic and intricate superspeciality, encompasses a broad spectrum of diseases affecting the joints, connective tissues, and immune system. These conditions, though prevalent, are often underrepresented in traditional medical education, leading to limited exposure for general physicians during their foundational training. However, with increasing awareness and advancements in diagnosis and treatment, rheumatology has emerged as a well-organized specialty with structured curricula and dedicated courses.

In clinical practice, patients presenting with musculoskeletal symptoms are frequently directed towards orthopedic consultations, sometimes missing underlying autoimmune or systemic conditions that require specialized care. Given the limited number of rheumatologists, it becomes imperative for general physicians to recognize and manage common rheumatologic conditions. This monograph aims to fill this gap by serving as a quick-reference guide, enabling physicians to grasp the fundamentals of rheumatology and address patient needs effectively.

Led by Dr G Narsimulu, Editor-in-Chief and an eminent figure in Indian rheumatology, this monograph also provides insights into recent advancements, offering an overview of essential rheumatologic management strategies. Dr Narsimulu's commitment to advancing rheumatology education and practice has been invaluable in shaping this resource. We extend our gratitude to the entire editorial team for their dedication and vision, as well as to the contributing authors, all experts in their respective fields. Additionally, we are grateful to the Association of Physicians of India (API) and the Indian College of Physicians (ICP) for their unwavering support in making this endeavor possible. May this monograph serve as a valuable resource for practitioners, reinforcing the strength of rheumatology within India's healthcare landscape.

Dr RK Singal
Dean, Indian College of Physicians
Academic wing of the Association of Physicians of India

Foreword

This monograph, *Bird's Eye View of Rheumatology*, is designed as a comprehensive, practical reference for physicians. Each chapter follows a structured format—covering introductions, clinical features, diagnostic criteria, and management options—making the content accessible and relevant to daily clinical practice. Treatment options are presented in a user-friendly table format, streamlining decision-making for busy practitioners.

The content of this monograph is crafted for practical application, and the contributions from seasoned experts across India reflect the latest standards in rheumatologic care. We are privileged to have Dr G Narsimulu as our Editor-in-Chief. A leader in the field, Dr Narsimulu has driven this project forward with dedication, ensuring the book's utility for the medical community. We also extend our heartfelt congratulations to the entire editorial team for their collective efforts in realizing this project, and we are confident that their contributions will enhance the daily practice of physicians who seek to expand their knowledge of rheumatologic conditions.

This monograph serves as a ready reckoner, equipping clinicians with essential knowledge to effectively manage patients and encouraging the integration of rheumatology into routine clinical practice.

Prof Rohini Honda
Past President, API
Senior Consultant Rheumatologist
Apollo Indroprastha Hospitals
New Delhi, India

Dear colleagues,

It is our pleasure to bring you this handy, concise, yet comprehensive book covering various important and clinically relevant topics. In *Bird's Eye View of Rheumatology*, the content has been carefully selected to address multiple aspects of rheumatology for primary healthcare providers on the frontline.

Understanding the complex and evolving concepts in rheumatology, we recognize that timely, concise, and accurate information is essential for effective patient care. This book is designed to bridge that need, offering an accessible, clear, and concise reference to support swift clinical decision-making and basic patient care for a range of rheumatic conditions. With topics covering pain syndromes, laboratory investigations, medications, and specific rheumatological diseases, this book will be a valuable resource for postgraduate and specialty trainees, as well as for physicians in both routine and emergency practice.

With contributions from leading experts in rheumatology, this handbook is a compilation of the latest evidence-based practices and practical insights, with easy-to-navigate sections including a clinical vignette at the end of each clinical topic.

We hope this ready reference becomes an indispensable resource in your clinical practice, empowering you to make informed decisions and enhancing the care you provide to your patients.

Thank you for your dedication to patient health and well-being.

Best wishes
The Editorial Team

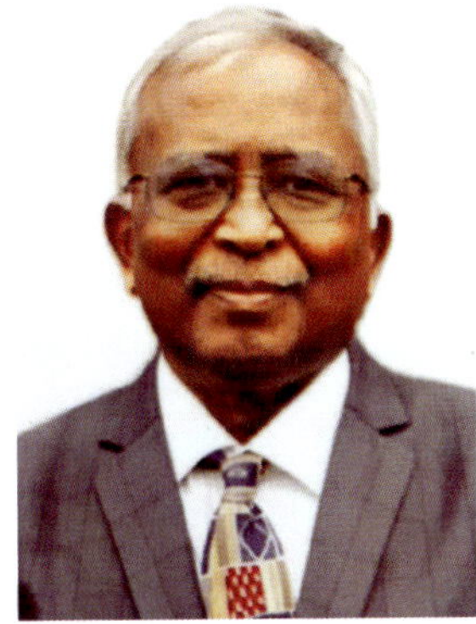

Gumdal Narsimulu MD, FICP, FIACM
President Elect
Association of Physicians of India
Sr. Consultant, Rheumatologist, GVN Medical Centre
Past President, Indian Rheumatology Association
Former Dean, ICP/API

Editor-in-Chief

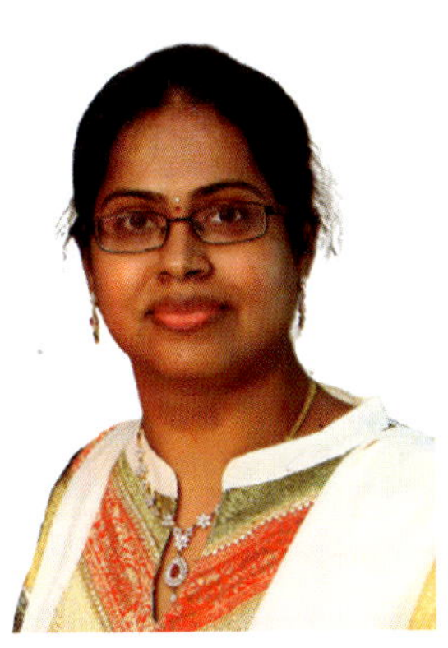

Keerthi Talari Bomamkanti MD, DM (Rheumatology)
Senior Consultant Rheumatologist
Yashoda Hospitals
Secunderabad, Hyderabad

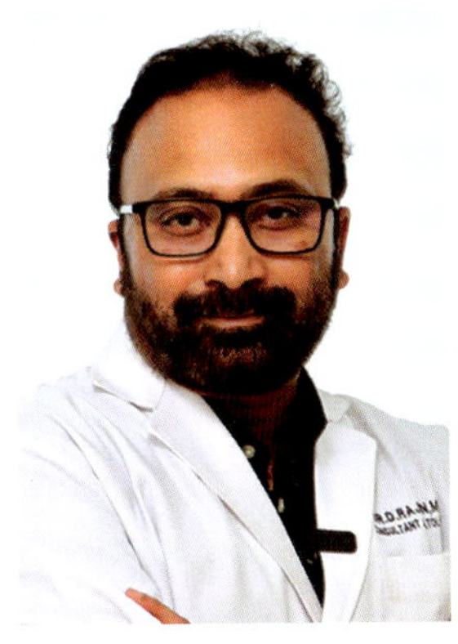

Rajkiran Dudam MD
Secretary Elect
Indian Rheumatology Association
Managing Director
HRC Hospitals
Hyderabad

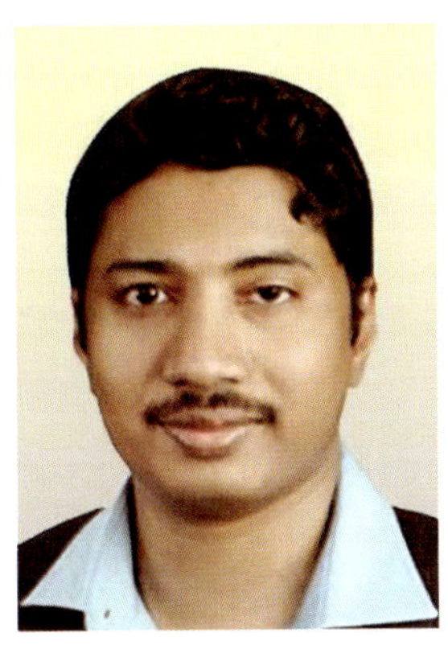

Irlapati Rajendra Varaprasad DM (Rheumatology), APLAR Fellow (UK)
Former Associate Profestsor, NIMS
Consultant Rheumatologist
Yashoda Hospitals
Somajiguda, Hyderabad

Reviewers List

Amirtha Gopalan MD, MRCP (UK), DrNB
Assistant Professor
Department of Clinical Immunology and
Rheumatology
Nizam's Institute of Medical Sciences
Hyderabad, India

Avanish Jha MD, DM
Associate Professor
Department of Clinical Immunology and
Rheumatology
Christian Medical College, Vellore, Tamil Nadu

Ramya Reddy Puligari MD, FIRH (KIMS)
Consultant Rheumatologist
HRC Hospital
Hyderabad, India

Rashmi Roongta MD, DM
Senior Resident
Department of Rheumatology
IPGMER and SSKM Hospital
Kolkata, West Bengal

Ritasman Baisya MD, DM
Assistant Professor
Department of Rheumatology
All India Institute of Medical Sciences
Kalyani, West Bengal

Shounak Ghosh MD, DrNB, MRCP
Consultant Rheumatologist
Calcutta Medical Research Institute
Kolkata, West Bengal

Adapa Ramakrishnam Naidu MD, DM (Rheumatology)
Head
Department of Clinical Immunology and Rheumatology
ESIC Medical College and Hospital
Hyderabad, India

Aditya Boney MBBS
Jr Medical Officer
Lourdes Hospital Post Graduate Institute of Medical Science and Research
Kochi, India

Ajaz Kariem Khan MD FACR FRCM
Director
Arthritis and Rheumatology Clinic of Kashmir
Srinagar, India

Akshay Parikh DM (Rheumatology)
Consultant Rheumatologist
AIG Hospitals
Hyderabad, India

Amirtha Gopalan MD, MRCP (UK), DrNB (Clinical Immunology and Rheumatology)
Assistant Professor
Nizam's Institute of Medical Sciences
Hyderabad, India

Amit Dua MBBS, DNB medicine, Fellow in Rheumatology
Consultant-Rheumatologist Dua's Clinic
Bilaspur, India

Aparna Reddy Sabbella MD (Medicine), DM (Rheumatology)
Consultant Rheumatologist
Sree Sanvi Oncology and Rheumatology Centre
Tirupati, india

Arindam Nandy Roy MD, Fellow Rheumatology (NIMS), FACR(USA)
Consultant Rheumatologist and Medical Director
Arthritis and Osteoporosis Clinic
Hyderabad, India

Arun Kumar Kedia MD, FICP
Consultant Physician
Lifeworth Hospital-Raipur
Assistant Professor, Department of Medicine
Raipur Institute of Medical Sciences
Raipur, India

Ashaq Hussain Parrey MD FACR
Assistant Professor
Department of Medicine and Rheumatology
Government Medical College
Srinagar, India

Bimlesh Dhar Pandey MD MRCP SCE (Rheumatology)
Director
Rheumatology Services
Fortis Hospital, Noida, India

Challa Madhuri MD (General Medicine), DM (Clinical Immunology and Rheumatology)
Assistant Professor
Nizam's Institute of Medical Sciences
Hyderabad, India

Col Arun Hegde MD, DNB (Rheumatology)
Professor (Medicine) and Rheumatologist
Commanding Officer
Military Hospital Belagavi
Belagavi, India

Durga Prasanna Misra DM, MRCP(UK), FRCP, MSc (Epidemiology)
Additional Professor
Clinical Immunology and Rheumatology
SGPGIMS, Lucknow, India

Emil J Thachil MD, DNB Rheumatology
Consultant Rheumatologist
Lourdes Hospital Post Graduate Institute of Medical Science and Research
Kochi, Ernakulam
Avitis Institute of Medical Sciences
Nemmara Palakkad, India

Gummadi Anjani MD (Pediatrics, PGIMER), DM (Pediatric Clinical Immunology and Rheumatology, PGIMER)
Consultant
Pediatric Rheumatologist and Immunologist
Ankura Hospitals for Women and Children
Hyderabad, India

Hema M MD, DM
Senior Assistant Professor
Department of Rheumatology
Government Stanley Medical College
Chennai, India

Himanshi Chaudhary MD, DM (Pediatric Clinical Immunology & Rheumatology)
Consultant Clinical Immunology and Pediatric Rheumatology
Alpha Superspeciality Clinics, Pune, India

Irlapati Rajendra Vara Prasad DM (Rheumatology), APLAR fellow (UCL,UK)
Consultant
Yashoda Hospital
Somajiguda, India

Jithin Mathew MBBS, MD, DM
Consultant
Clinical Immunology and Rheumatology
Yashoda Hospital
Hitec City, Hyderabad, India

Kavitha Mohanasundaram MD, DM, SCE
Consultant Rheumatologist
Kauvery Hospitals
Radial Road, Chennai

KV Kishore Babu MD, DM
Consultant Rheumatologist
Shine Rheumatology Centre
Nellore, India

Kavyasree Sunil MD, DrNB Resident
Senior Resident
Department of Rheumatology
Topiwala National Medical College
Mumbai, India

Keerthi Talari Bomamkanti MD, DM (Rheumatology)
Senior Consultant Rheumatologist
Yashoda Hospitals
Secunderabad, Hyderabad, India

Kshiti Rai MD (Resident Medicine)
Government Medical College
Kozhikode, India

Kushagra Gupta MD (Fellowship in Rheumatology)
Consultant Rheumatologist
Joint and Autoimmune Clinic
Gupta Medical Centre, Hisar, India

Lalit Duggal MD FRCP
Chairman, Department of Rheumatology and Clinical Immunology
Sir Ganga Ram Hospital
New Delhi, India

Lt Col Sankar MD, DM (Rheumatology)
Classified Specialist (Medicine) and Rheumatologist
Army Hospital Research and Referral
Delhi Cantt, India

M Harish Kumar MD DNB MNAMS, Trainde in Rheumatology (NIMS), PG Diploma in MSK USG (UCAM, Spain)
Classified Specialist Medicine and Rheumatology
12 Air Force Hospital, Gorakhpur, India

Madhuri HR DM (Rheumatology)
Senior Consultant Rheumatologist
Star Hospitals
Financial district, Hyderabad, India

Manisha Ashwin Daware MD, DNB (General Medicine), Fellowship in Rheumatology
Consultant Rheumatology
Manipal Hospital
Whitefield, Bengaluru

Mohit Goyal MD, FRCP, FACR
Consultant Rheumatologist
CARE Pain and Arthritis Centre
Udaipur, India

Muppalla Mowlika MD (General Medicine), DrNB (Rheumatology Resident)
ESIC Medical College and Superspeciality Hospital
Hyderabad, India

N Kavya Devi MD, DM (Rheumatology)
Consultant Rheumatologist
Anvitha Arthritis and Rheumatology Centre
Vijayawada, india

NV Jayachandran MD, DNB (Rheumatology), FRCP (Edin)
Professor
Department of Medicine and Rheumatologist
Government Medical College
Kozhikode, India

Nilesh Nolkha MBBS, MD, DM (Rheumatology)
Rheumatology Incharge
DNB guide and Senior Consultant
Rheumatologist
Topiwala National Medical College and BYL
Nair Charitable Hospital
Nirjara Multispeciality Clinics
Mumbai

P Damodaram DM
Consultant Rheumatologist
Shubodaya Rheumatology Hospital
Tirupati, India

P Sree Sanjay MBBS
Shubodaya Rheumatology Hospital
Tirupati, india

PD Rath MD, FACR, FRCP (Edin), FRCP (Glasgow) FNIMS, FRCM, GCPR (Aus) Diploma MSK USG (UCAM Spain)
Senior Director and Head
Department of Rheumatology
Max Super Speciality Hospital
Saket, Panchsheel, India

Parthajit Das MD, FRCP (London), FRCP (Edin), CCT-Rheum, MSC (Sports Medicine)
Consultant Rheumatologist
Asian Institute of Immunology and
Rheumatology
Kolkata, India

Phani Kumar D MD, DM
Additional Professor
Nizam's Institute of Medical Sciences
Hyderabad, India

Pothireddy Mohith Kumar Reddy
MD (DrNB Rheumatology)
Senior Resident
KIMS Hospitals
Secunderabad, Hyderabad, India

Pratyusha Rajavarapu MD, DM (Rheumatology)
Consultant Rheumatologist
Pratyusha Rheumatology care
Assistant Professor
Department of Rheumatology
NRIMC, Guntur, India

Pravin Hissaria MBBS, MD, DM, FRCPA, FRACP
Clinical Immunologist and Immunopathologist
Head of the Unit
Clinical Immunology and Allergy
Royal Adelaide Hospital
Adelaide, South Australia

Pravin Patil MRCP (UK), FRCP (Edin), CCT (Rheum)
Consultant Rheumatologist
Pune Rheumatology Center
Maharashtra, India

Ramya Janardana MD, Fellowship in Rheumatology
Professor
Department of Clinical Immunology and
Rheumatology
St John's Hospital, Bengaluru, India

Ramya Reddy Puligari MD, FIRH (KIMS)
Consultant Rheumatologist
HRC Hospital, Hyderabad, India

Ranjan Gupta MD (General Medicine), DM (Clinical Immunology)
Additional Professor
Department of Rheumatology
All India Institute of Medical Sciences (AIIMS)
New Delhi, india

Sai Sunil B
Senior Resident
KIMS, KIIT University,
Bhubaneshwar, India

Sakir Ahmed MD, DM, MAMS
Associate Professor
KIMS, KIIT University, Bhubaneshwar, India

Saranya C MD (General Medicine), DM (Rheumatology)
Professor
Department of Rheumatology
Saveetha Medical College and Hospital
Chennai, India

Sarath Chandra Mouli Veeravalli
MD, FRCP (London)
Clinical Director
Department of Rheumatology and Clinical Immunology
KIMS Hospitals
Secunderabad, Hyderabad, India

Shabina Habibi DM (Rheumatology), MRCP (London)
Consultant Rheumatology and Lead
Osteoporosis and Fracture Liaison Services
Queens Hospital, Romford, UK

Sham Santhanam MD, DM, MRCP (UK), FRCP (Edin.)
Senior Consultant
Rheumatologist
Kauvery Hospital Alwarpet
Chennai, India

Shruti Sripati MRCP, SCE (Rheumatology)
Consultant Rheumatologist
KIMS Sunshine Hospital
Begumpet, Hyderabad, India

Shweta Agarwal MBBS, MD (Medicine)
Professor
Department of Medicine and Integral Institute
of Medical Sciences and Research Integral University
Lucknow, India

Silas Supragya Nelson MD, Fellowship in Rheumatology (NIMS)
Consultant Rheumatologist
Professor
Department of Medicine
Incharge Division of Rheumatology
NSCB Medical College
Jabalpur, India

Sirisha K MD, DM
Consultant Rheumatologist
ISHA Superspecialty Clinics
Tirupati, India

Sneha Babu
Junior Resident
Department of Internal Medicine
Government Stanley Medical College
Chennai, India

Sowmya Kotha DM (Clinical Immunology and Rheumatology)
Assistant Professor
Nizam's Institute of Medical Sciences
Hyderabad, India

Spoorthy Kothapalli
Consultant Rheumatologist
KIMS, Kondapur
Spoorthy Rheumatology and Kidney Care, KPHB
Hyderabad, India

Sravan Kumar Appani MD, DM (Rheumatology)
Consultant Rheumatologist
Rishi Rheumatology Centre
Karimnagar, India

Sreejitha KS MBBS, MD (General Medicine), DM (Clinical Immunology and Rheumatology)
Consultant Rheumatologist
Manipal Hospital
Old Airport Road, Bangalore

Srinivasa C MD DM
Consultant Rheumatologist
Fortis Hospital, Bannerghatta Road
Bangalore, India

Srujana Arekal MD, DM (Rheumatology)
Consultant Rheumatologist
Jeevan Rayalaseema Rheumatology Centre
Medicover Hospitals
Kurnool, India

Sunitha Kayidhi MD (General Medicine), DM (Rheumatology)
Senior Consultant Rheumatologist
Continental Hospitals, Hyderabad, India

Sureja Nayan Patel MD, DM
Consultant Rheumatologist
Star Hospitals (Banjara Hills)
Hyderabad, India

Tejaswee MD
Senior Resident (DrNB) Rheumatology
Max Hospital, Saket, New Delhi, India

VA Deepika Ponnuru MD (Medicine) DM (Rheumatology)
Consultant Rheumatologist
Manipal Hospitals, Vijayawada

VN Nagaprabhu DNB (Rheumatology)
Consultant Rheumatologist
Sakthi Rheumatology Centre Pvt Ltd
Coimbatore, Tamil Nadu, India

Velammal P DNB (Medicine), MNAMS
Professor
Department of Internal Medicine
PSGIMS&R
Coimbatore, Tamil Nadu, India

Vijaya Prasanna Parimi MD DM
(Rheumatology)
Senior Consultant Rheumatologist
ESIC Medical College and Super Speciality Hospital
Hyderabad, India

Vikramraj K Jain MD (Medicine), DM (Clinical
Immunology, JIPMER), RhMSUS (ACR, USA)
Consultant Immunologist and Rheumatologist
Bhagwan Mahaveer Jain Hospital and Optima
Superspeciality Rheumatology Hospital
Bengaluru, India

Vinod Ravindran MD, CCT, FRCP
Consultant Rheumatologist
Department of Rheumatology
Centre for Rheumatology
Calicut, Kerala, India
Adjunct Professor of Medicine
Kasturba Medical College
Manipal Academy of Higher Education
Manipal, Karnataka, India

Contents

Section IV: Crystal Arthropathies

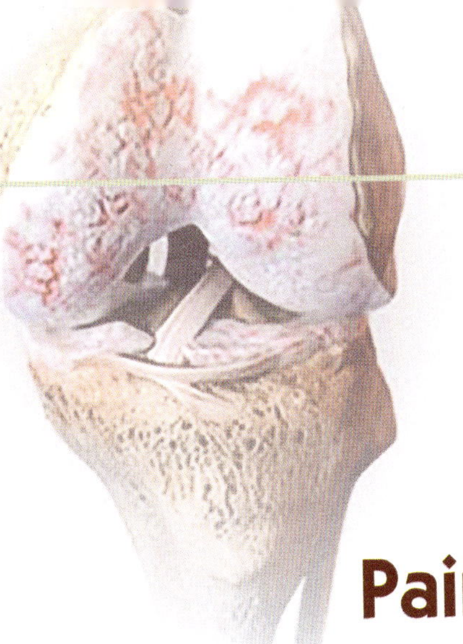

Pain Syndromes

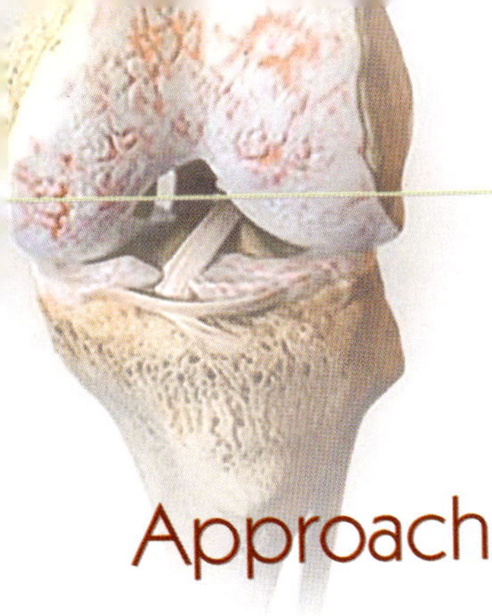

Approach to Arthritis

Arindam Nandy Roy

The term "arthritis" refers to the swelling of a joint or joints associated with pain, heat, tenderness and limitation of movements unlike "arthralgia" which means joint pain without any abnormalities on examination. Arthritis is the pathological feature in over 200 rheumatic disease conditions and also can be the initial presentation of diseases such as endocrinopathies and cancer.

The evaluation of arthritis should determine whether it is articular or periarticular (bursitis, tendinitis, etc.), inflammatory (presence of systemic symptoms, early morning stiffness of >1 hr and signs of joint inflammation) or noninflammatory (absence of above features), and the number and pattern of involvement of joints (Fig. 1.1 and Box 1.1).

Following is a stepwise approach to patients with arthritis:

Step 1: Initial assessment, which involves:

1. *Medical history:* Collecting information about the patient's symptoms, such as joint pain or stiffness, swelling or redness, limited mobility or function, duration and pattern of symptoms. Ask about family history of arthritis or other autoimmune

Musculoskeletal pain
   Articular
      Noninflammatory
         Osteoarthritis
         Hypothyroidism

      Inflammatory
         Monoarthritis
            Gout,Septic arthritis/TB arthritis

         Oligoarthritis
            Gout, SpA, PsA

         Polyarthritis
            RA, SLE, PsA

Fig 1.1: Approach to a patient with polyarticular pain. SpA: Spondyloarthritis; RA: Rheumatoid arthritis; TB: Tuberculosis; SLE: Systemic lupus erythematosus; PsA: Psoriatic arthritis (*Adapted from* Handa: Clinical Rheumatology, 2021)

Box 1.1: Pattern recognition in arthritis (*Adapted from* Handa: Clinical Rheumatology, 2021)

Mode of onset
Acute: Septic arthritis, reactive arthritis, viral arthritis, gout or trauma
Insidious: Rheumatoid arthritis, spondyloarthritis, osteoarthritis

Duration
Acute (lasting <6 weeks): Viral arthritis
Chronic (lasting >6 weeks): Rheumatoid arthritis

Number of affected joints
Monoarthritis (single joint involvement): Septic arthritis, tubercular arthritis, gout
Oligoarthritis (2–4 joints involvement): Gout, juvenile idiopathic arthritis, spondyloarthritis
Polyarthritis (≥5 joints involvement): Rheumatoid arthritis, systemic lupus erythematosus

Distribution
Symmetrical (rheumatoid arthritis) or asymmetrical (gout)
Lower limbs (spondyloarthritis) versus upper limbs (rheumatoid arthritis)
Small joints (rheumatoid arthritis) versus large joints (spondyloarthritis)
Specific joints (distal interphalangeal joints in osteoarthritis)

Extra-articular features
Fever as in adult onset Still's disease
Mucocutaneous lesions as in systemic lupus erythematosus
Eye involvement as in spondyloarthritis
Nodules as in tophaceous gout

Sequence of involvement
Intermittent arthritis as in palindromic rheumatism
Migratory arthritis as in rheumatic fever
Additive arthritis as in rheumatoid arthritis

   diseases, previous joint injuries or surgeries, current medications and supplements, lifestyle habits (e.g., exercise, diet, smoking).

2. *Physical examination:* Inspecting the affected joints for swelling or redness, warmth or tenderness, deformities or contractures. Assess joint mobility and function for range of motion, strength, stability, gait and balance. Check for extra-articular features (e.g., skin rashes, eye inflammation)

3. *Identifying the type of arthritis:* Based on the history and physical examination, consider the possibility of osteoarthritis (wear and tear), rheumatoid arthritis (autoimmune), psoriatic arthritis (associated with psoriasis), other types of arthritis (e.g., gout, lupus, ankylosing spondylitis).

This initial assessment helps the physician to develop a preliminary diagnosis, identify potential red flags (e.g., signs of infection or malignancy), determine the need for further diagnostic testing and begin developing a treatment plan.

Step 2: Diagnostic tests

1. Diagnostic tests to confirm the type of arthritis and rule out other conditions like rheumatoid factor (RF), anti-citrullinated protein antibodies (anti-CCP), antinuclear antibody (ANA), erythrocyte sedimentation rate (ESR), C-reactive protein (CRP), complete blood count (CBC), blood chemistry tests (e.g., liver and kidney function), etc.

2. Imaging studies like X-rays to assess joint damage and degeneration, USG to evaluate joint inflammation and synovitis, magnetic resonance imaging (MRI) to assess joint and soft tissue inflammation and computed tomography (CT) scan to evaluate bone and joint damage.

3. Joint aspiration for synovial fluid analysis for inflammation, infection, or crystals.
4. Other tests like urinalysis to rule out kidney disease, stool test to rule out gastrointestinal bleeding and bone density test (DXA) to assess osteoporosis risk.

Step 3: Developing a treatment plan based on the diagnosis and individual patient needs.

1. Non-pharmacological interventions include patient education (understanding the condition, treatment options, and self-management), lifestyle modifications (exercise, weight management, stress management, smoking cessation), assistive devices (canes, walkers, splints, orthotics) and physical therapy (range of motion, strengthening, flexibility).
2. Pharmacological interventions include analgesics, corticosteroids (e.g., prednisolone), DMARDs (e.g., methotrexate, hydroxychloroquine), biologics: targeting specific molecules (e.g., TNF-alpha, IL-17), target synthetic DMARDs (e.g., tofacitinib), disease-modifying osteoarthritis drugs (DMOADs), etc.
3. Surgical interventions include joint replacement (e.g., hip, knee, shoulder), joint fusion, osteotomy (bone realignment), soft tissue procedures (e.g., tendon repair), etc.

Step 4: Involves monitoring and follow-up to assess treatment effectiveness, adjust the treatment plan as needed, and monitor for potential side effects.

1. *Regular assessments:* Schedule regular appointments (e.g., every 3–6 months). Assess symptoms, functional status, and quality of life and evaluate treatment effectiveness and adjust plan as needed.
2. *Disease activity monitoring:* Use standardized measures (e.g., DAS28, CDAI) to assess disease activity and monitor for signs of disease flare or progression.
3. *Side effect monitoring:* Monitor for potential side effects of medications (e.g., liver function, kidney function) and assess for signs of infection, malignancy, or other complications.
4. *Lifestyle and behavioural modifications:* Encourage ongoing lifestyle modifications (e.g., exercise, weight management) and address behavioural factors (e.g., stress, smoking) that may impact disease activity.
5. *Patient education and empowerment:* Provide ongoing patient education and support and encourage self-management and empowerment.
   The approach to arthritis is predominantly clinical and relies heavily on history and physical examination. Patient education and empowerment are crucial for successful management.

FURTHER READING

1. Handa R. Bedside approach to musculoskeletal complaints. In: Handa: Clinical Rheumatology.1st ed 2021.p.1–8.
2. Imboden J. Approach to the patient with arthritis. In:Imboden JB, Stone JH, Hellmann DB ed. Current Rheumatology Diagnosis & Treatment.2nd ed. Tata McGraw-Hill 2009:p.32–41.

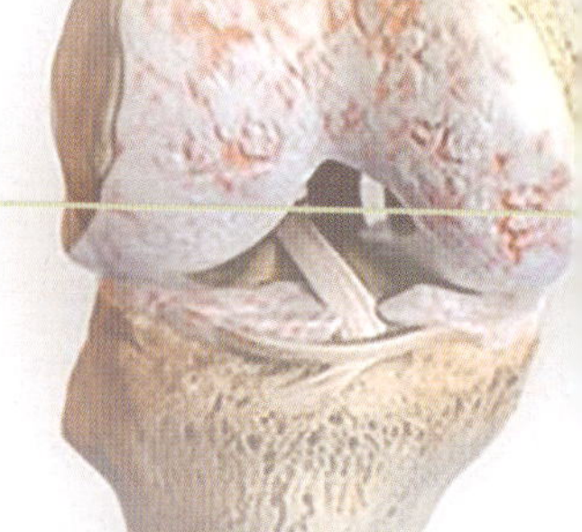

Low Back Pain

Ashaq Hussain Parrey, Ajaz Kariem Khan

INTRODUCTION

The World Health Organisation defines low back pain (LBP) as, any pain in back between the lower edge of the ribs and the gluteal folds. Lower back pain is the number one cause of disability worldwide and most prevalent chronic pain syndrome. The LBP is classified on the basis of duration into acute LBP (less than 4 weeks), subacute (4 to 12 weeks) and chronic (more than 12 weeks) of duration. It is estimated that up to 84 percent of adults have low back pain at some point of time in their life. For the purpose of management, the LBP is classified into two categories: Mechanical inflammatory.

Mechanical Low Back Pain

Mechanical back pain is typically caused by anatomic or physiological abnormality of spinal joints, discs, vertebrae or soft tissue. The pain is generally aggravated by activity and upright posture and is partially or completely relieved by rest. Majority of patients 95 to 99% with LBP have mechanical back pain. These patients improve in a few days to a few weeks, usually less than 4 weeks and the major contribution for this pain is musculoskeletal in origin. The pain may or may not be associated with radiculopathy. Radiculopathy refers to symptoms or impairments related to a spinal nerve root, and 90 percent of radiculopathies originate from the L5 and S1 nerve roots. Sciatica is a nonspecific term used to describe a variety of leg or back symptoms, usually refers to a sharp or burning pain radiating down from the buttock along the course of the sciatic nerve (the posterior or lateral aspect of the leg up to the foot or ankle). Less than 1 percent of patients with mechanical LBP have a serious underlying cause like cauda equina syndrome, metastatic cancer, and spinal infection or vertebral osteomyelitis.

Inflammatory Back Pain (IBP)

Inflammatory back pain" typically exhibits at least four of the following five features. Age of onset less than 40 years, insidious onset, improvement with exercise, no improvement with rest, pain at night (with improvement upon arising). The inflammatory back pain is typically associated with morning stiffness that lasts for more than 30 min and the pain is often worse during the second half of night. Approximately 3 to 6% of patients with low back pain have inflammatory back pain and 9 to 15% of those with IBP (0.9 to 1.5% patients with LBP) have axial spondyloarthropathy. The hallmark of

IBP is an excellent response to nonsteroidal anti-inflammatory drugs (NSAIDs). The causes of inflammatory back pain include inflammatory conditions like ankylosing spondylitis, psoriatic arthritis, reactive arthritis, inflammatory bowel disease related spondyloarthropathy and infections like Brucella and tubercular discitis.

DIAGNOSIS

The diagnosis of low back pain is made on the basis of history of illness, examination and imaging as described below.

History Taking in Patient with Low Back Pain

- **Onset and duration:** When did the pain start. Is it acute (less than 4 weeks) subacute (4 to 12 weeks or chronic (more than 12 weeks).
- **Location:** Where is the pain located, does it radiate to the legs, hips, or elsewhere.
- **Character of pain:** Is the pain sharp, dull, throbbing, or burning? Is it constant or intermittent?
- **Aggravating and relieving factors:** What activities or positions worsen or alleviate the pain.
- **Associated symptoms:** Any numbness, tingling, weakness, or bowel/bladder dysfunction.
- **Previous episodes:** Has the patient experienced similar pain before?
- **Medical history:** Any history of trauma, surgery, infections, or underlying conditions like arthritis or osteoporosis.

Examination of a Patient with Low Back Pain

- **Inspection:** Observe posture, gait, and any obvious deformities or asymmetry.
- **Palpation:** Check for tenderness, muscle spasms, or trigger points in the lower back.
- **Range of motion (ROM):** Assess the range of motion in the lumbar spine (flexion, extension, lateral bending, and rotation).
- **Neurological examination:** Test muscle strength in the lower extremities.
- **Sensation:** Check for sensory deficits using light touch, pinprick, or vibration.
- **Reflexes:** Test deep tendon reflexes (e.g., patellar and Achilles reflexes).
- **Straight leg raise (SLR) test:** Helps to identify nerve root irritation, often due to herniated discs.
- **Special tests:** Depending on symptoms, additional tests like the Patrick's test (FABER) for sacroiliac joint issues or the Thomas test for hip flexor tightness might be performed to assess the flexibility of the iliopsoas and other hip flexor muscles, which can contribute to restricted hip extension or lower back pain.

Red Flags in Low Back Pain

- Severe, unrelenting pain (especially at night)
- Neurological deficits (e.g., foot drop, saddle anesthesia)
- History of cancer or unexplained weight loss
- Fever or history of intravenous drug use (suggesting infection)
- Recent trauma (especially in the elderly)
- Osteoporosis (risk of compression fractures).

Diagnostic Tests in Low Back Pain

- **Imaging:** Usually reserved for cases where red flags are present or if conservative treatment fails.
- **X-rays:** May show fractures, degenerative changes, or alignment issues.
- **MRI:** Useful for identifying disc herniations, spinal stenosis, tumors, or infections.
- **CT scan:** Often used when MRI is contraindicated.
- **Blood tests:** In cases where infection, inflammation, or malignancy is suspected, tests like ESR, CRP, and complete blood count (CBC) may be ordered.
- **Electromyography (EMG) and nerve conduction studies:** If there's suspicion of nerve involvement, these tests can help assess the electrical activity of muscles and nerves.

Thus, meticulous history taking, clinical examination and appropriate diagnostic testing will aid diagnosis.

FURTHER READING

1. Diagnosis and treatment of low back pain: a joint clinical practice guideline from the American College of Physicians and the American Pain Society. Chou R, Qaseem A, Snow V, Casey D, Cross JT Jr, Shekelle P, Owens DK, Clinical Efficacy Assessment Subcommittee of the American College of Physicians, American College of Physicians, American Pain Society Low Back Pain Guidelines Panel Ann Intern Med. 2007;147(7):478.
2. What can history and physical examination tell us about low back pain? Deyo RA, Rainville J, Kent DL JAMA. 1992;268(6):760. Health Services Research and Development Field Program, Seattle Veterans Affair Medical Center, WA.
3. Sieper J, et al. New criteria for inflammatory back pain in patients with chronic back pain: A real patient exercise by experts from the Assessment of Spondyloarthritis International Society (ASAS). Ann Rheum Dis. 2009;68(6):784.

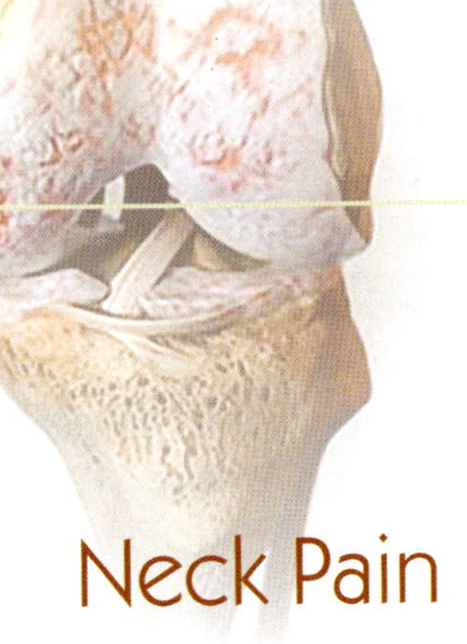

Neck Pain

Ramya Reddy Puligari

INTRODUCTION

Neck pain is frequently evaluated by rheumatologists, with mechanical issues being the most common cause. It can stem from problems with the spine, surrounding soft tissues, the spinal cord, nerve roots, or even be referred from other organs. Most neck pain is non-serious and nonspecific. In older adults, it is more prevalent due to degeneration of facet joints and intervertebral disc collapse. For younger individuals, it is crucial to consider non-mechanical causes, as inflammatory arthritis, although less common.

Causes

Neck pain can lead to significant disability, varying from mild discomfort to severe, debilitating pain. Causes can range from benign muscular strains to serious conditions like fractures, autoimmune disorders, neoplastic diseases, and infections.

The most frequent atraumatic cause is cervical strain, often due to spasm of the cervical muscles from physical stressors like poor posture, improper sleeping habits, or injuries. Symptoms may persist for up to 6 weeks, and alternative diagnoses should be explored if symptoms are atypical or prolonged. Cervical spondylosis, results from disc degeneration and presents with pain and stiffness during neck movement. Intervertebral disc desiccation can lead to osteophyte formation, compressing nerve roots and causing mechanical pain. Whiplash, a common traumatic cause, results from rapid neck flexion-extension and can cause persistent pain even when imaging shows no structural abnormalities.

Neuropathic causes include cervical radiculopathy from degenerative changes like foraminal stenosis or herniated discs, leading to arm pain, sensory changes, and possible motor weakness. Cervical myelopathy, caused by spinal cord dysfunction from spondylosis and canal narrowing, is also a key concern.

In rheumatology, cervical spine pathology affects over half of patients with rheumatoid arthritis, increasing their risk of severe complications like spinal cord impingement. Ankylosing spondylitis heightens the risk of fractures from even minor trauma. Myofascial pain features trigger points in taut muscle bands that produce referred pain when pressed, while fibromyalgia is characterized by excessively tender soft tissue sites (Tables 3.1 and 3.2).

Table 3.1: Rheumatological disorders commonly involving neck	
Rheumatoid arthritis	C1–C2 (atlantoaxial) subluxation, basilar invagination, pannus formation of odontoid process
Ankylosing spondylitis	C1–C2 subluxation, ankylosis, C5–C6 fracture
Juvenile idiopathic arthritis	C1–C2 subluxation, C2–C3 fusion, fusion of apophyseal joints
Osteoarthritis	C5–C7 spondylosis
Diffuse idiopathic skeletal hyperostosis (DISH)	Anterior longitudinal ligament ossification
Polymyalgia rheumatica	Pain and stiffness in neck with constitutional symptoms
Polymyositis	Flexor muscle weakness
Fibromyalgia	C2, C5–C7 tender points
Takayasu aortoarteritis	Carotidynia
Sarcoidosis	Cervical myelopathy, intramedullary granulomas

Table 3.2: Other causes of neck pain	
Non-traumatic	Spondylosis, neck strain, myelopathy, radiculopathy, disc prolapse
Traumatic	Whiplash, disc herniation, cervical fracture
Neoplastic	Metastasis, multiple myeloma, ciant cell tumor, osteoblastoma, osteochondroma
Infectious	Discitis, osteomyelitis, meningitis, epidural abscess, herpes zoster
Neurological	Transverse myelitis, brachial plexitis, ALS, GBS, CRPS, peripheral entrapment
Endocrinological	Paget's disease, osteoporosis, PTH disorders
Miscellaneous and referred pain	AV fistula and malformation, syringomyelia, thoracic outlet syndrome, oesophagitis, pancoast tumor, vascular dissection, angina, aortic dissection, thyroiditis, peritonsillar or retropharyngeal abscess

APPROACH

Accurate clinical history is crucial for initial evaluation. Distinguishing between acute and chronic symptoms, and identifying neuropathic versus non-neuropathic symptoms, helps gauge urgency. Vigilance for red flags during history and physical examination is essential, as these may signal the need for urgent testing and intervention (Box 3.1).

Box 3.1: Red flag signs necessitating immediate investigation
• Fever, weight loss, nausea and vomiting
• Severe headache, visual loss, photo or phonophobia, ataxia, incontinence
• Neck stiffness, severe tenderness, torticollis (cervical dystonia)
• History of malignancy, immunosuppression, Intravenous drug abuse, recent surgery or instrumentation
• Ripping, tearing sensaton in the neck: Vascular dissection
• Concurrent chest pain, shortness of breath, diaphoresis: Ischemic heart disease
• Worsening/persisting inflammatory pain, raised ESR/CRP/leucocyte count

Mechanical musculoskeletal pain is typically dull, deep, and aching, with occasional sharp exacerbations. Comparison of active and passive range of motion is useful for differentiating articular and non-articular pain. Pain that deviates from this pattern, such as shooting or electrical pain, may indicate neural involvement.

Rapidly progressive neuropathic symptoms require more comprehensive evaluation. Even in the absence of acute symptoms, watch for myelopathic signs, including increased muscle tone, fasciculations, clonus, hyperreflexia, and the Babinski reflex. Provocative tests, such as the Spurling's test, are highly specific and sensitive, particularly when assessing for radiculopathy. When there's suspicion of instability or fracture in the cervical spine, performing provocative tests can be dangerous.

Imaging and Management

Plain radiographs can reveal osteophytes and disc narrowing, indicating disc degeneration. To assess atlantoaxial joint subluxation in rheumatoid arthritis (RA), open mouth and lateral flexion/extension radiographs are used. For suspected tumors, infections, or root impingement, MRI is more precise and provides the best technique for identifying the cause and location. Management should primarily target the underlying cause, whether it is inflammatory, infectious, or myelopathic—the latter often necessitating urgent surgical decompression. Most mechanical issues typically improve with time and conservative treatment.

Key Points

- Identify and address "red flags" and "yellow flags" (risk factors for chronic pain) early in treatment.
- Distinguish between neuropathic and non-neuropathic cervicalgia to guide investigations and treatment.
- Atlanto-axial subluxation in rheumatic conditions can indicate severe disease activity early management prevents complications.
- Early detection of systemic inflammatory illnesses through diagnostic work-up allows for timely treatment and prevents progression.

FURTHER READING

1. Loh, Raina Hui Wen BMed MD, MMED (FM)[1]; Leong, Adriel Zhijie MBBS, MMED (Surg)[2]; Lwin, Sein MMed (Gen Surg), FRCS (Surg Neuro)[3]; Goh, Lee Gan MMed, FCFP1. An approach to neck pain in primary care. Singapore Medical Journal 65(6):p 348–53, June 2024.|DOI: 10.4103/singaporemedj.SMJ-2021-288
2. Oberstein EM, Carpintero M, Hopkins A. Neck pain from a rheumatologic perspective. Phys Med Rehabil Clin N Am. 2011 Aug; 22(3):485–502, ix. doi: 10.1016/j.pmr.2011.02.009. Epub 2011 Jun 15. PMID: 21824589.

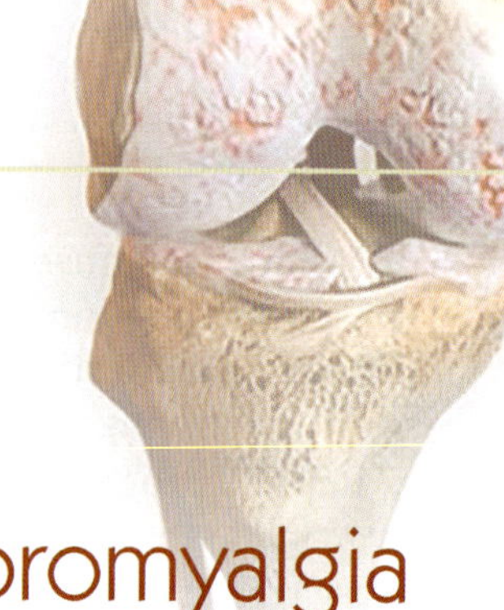

Fibromyalgia

Aparna Reddy Sabbella

INTRODUCTION

Fibromyalgia (FM) remains one of the most puzzling, mysterious medical conditions. It is known for its chronic persistent widespread pain, which is of predominantly non-inflammatory type. The non-musculoskeletal symptoms are fatigue, cognitive symptoms, mood disorders, sleep disturbances. In terms of prevalence FM ranks third next to lumbar pain, osteoarthritis. The important limiting factor in management of FM is lack of objective markers.

Fibromyalgia is characterised by central sensitisation along with small fibre neuropathy. The pain driving immunoglobulins act on the satellite glial cells present in the dorsal root ganglia. The individuals who exhibit increased intensity of symptoms may have demonstrable neuroinflammation. The titre of anti-satellite glial cell IgG correlated with disease severity in a study. FM is associated with changes in neurotransmitters of the brain.

Clinical Features and Diagnosis

The clinical features of FM are listed in Table 4.1. The diagnosis of FM relies on the clinical judgement of the treating physician.

The revised American College of Rheumatology criteria diagnosis of FM:

A patient who meets the following three criteria:
1. The patient scores $\geq$7 on the widespread pain index (WPI) and $\geq$5 on the symptom severity (SS) scale, or the patient scores 3–6 on the WPI and 9 on the SS scale.
2. The patient's symptoms have been present at a similar level for at least 3 months.
3. The patient does not have a disorder that would otherwise explain their pain.

The WPI, if a patient has had pain during the past week. Assign one point for each area. The total score will be between 0 and 19.

The symptom severity scale evaluates
1. The severity of three specific symptoms plus.
2. The severity of somatic symptoms in general.
The total score will be between 0 and 12.

Table 4.1: Clinical features of fibromyalgia	
Symptoms	*Description*
Pain	• Generalized (head-to-toes) • Described in terms of neuropathic pain, paresthesias
Fatigue	• Physical • Mental
Sleep disturbances	• Insomnia • Frequent awakening • Non-restoring sleep
Psychiatric symptoms	• Anxiety • Depression • Post-traumatic stress disorder
Cognitive dysfunctions	• Concentration difficulties • Memory deficits
Autonomic disturbances	• Blurred vision, photophobia and xerophthalmia • Feeling of instability • Xerostomia • Variations in responses to cold at the extremities (including Raynaud phenomenon) • Orthostatic hypotension
Stiffness	• Morning stiffness not exceeding 60 min
Regional pain syndromes	• Migraine or headache • Stomach ache or dyspepsia • Abdominal pain or irritable bowel syndrome • Dysmenorrhoea • Vulvodynia • Dysuria
Hypersensitivity to external stimuli	• Hypersensitivity to light, odours and sounds • Chemical sensitivity

Treatment

Non-pharmacological

The treatment is based on major symptoms and is individualized. The active therapies proposed are:

1. Muscle stretching exercises
2. Mind-body techniques
3. Resistance training
4. Aerobic exercises
5. Pilates
6. Swimming
7. Whole body vibration
8. Tai chi
9. **Nutritional interventions:** Olive oil, ancient grains, low-calorie diets, gluten-free options, and Mediterranean diets, supplementation with acetyl-carnitine, coenzyme Q10, chlorella green algae, and vitamins C and E.

Probiotics: The role of gut flora as a causative agent in FM and chronic fatigue syndrome have been proposed. Anxiety levels were likely to be decreased by *Lactobacillus* sp. A significant reduction in inflammatory markers was seen with *Bifidobacterium infantis*.

10. Psychotherapy
11. Cognitive behavioural therapy
12. Acupuncture
13. Electrophysical agents: transcranial magnetic stimulation, transcranial direct current stimulation to the motor cortex (M1) or dorsolateral prefrontal cortex best alleviates pain.

- Hyperbaric oxygen therapy with its neuroplasticity effects is another possible strategy of treatment.

Pharmacological

The medications proposed for treatment of fibromyalgia and mechanism of action is shown in Table 4.2. In situations of inadequate response, a combination could be tried.

Combination of different drugs:

1. Antidepressants (such as tricyclic antidepressants—amitriptyline and nortriptyline or serotonin norepinephrine reuptake inhibitors—duloxetine, venlafaxine and milnacipran) with anticonvulsants (such as gabapentin or pregabalin).
2. Opioid analgesics (such as oxycodone or tramadol) are not to be used regularly in view of its addictive potential although may give symptomatic benefit.

Table 4.2: Pharmacological management of fibromyalgia		
Medication	*Medication category*	*Mechanism of action*
Nortriptyline and amitriptyline	Tricyclic antidepressants	Increase serotonin and norepinephrine levels, thereby help in reducing anxiety, depression, chronic pain
Milnacipran, venlafaxine and duloxetine	Serotonin norepinephrine reuptake inhibitors (SNRIs)	Increase the neurotransmitter levels, thereby improving anxiety, depression, chronic pain and fibromyalgia
Pregabalin, gabapentin and topiramate	Anticonvulsant/ antiepileptic drugs	Modulate neurotransmitter release, reducing neuropathic pain
Tramadol and oxycodone	Opioid analgesics	They bind to opioid receptors, reduce pain perception
Mirtazapine, trazodone, amisulpiride, quetiapine	Atypical antidepressants	They help in treatment of depression, sleep disorders, anxiety in fibromyalgia
Cannabis	Cannabis and cannabinoids	They help in conditions of chronic pain, reducing inflammation
NSAIDs and lidocaine	Non-opioid analgesics	These block production of prostaglandin and reduce pain
Quetiapine, olanzapine, Acetyl-L-carnitine	Antipsychotic drugs	These are helpful in the treatment of sleep disorders and anxiety

3. Zolpidem or trazodone with antidepressants.
4. Cyclobenzaprine or tizanidine (muscle relaxants) with antidepressants.

Conclusion

- Fibromyalgia remains a disease with either under diagnosis or misdiagnosis, due to lack of sufficient objective markers.
- The quality of life can be improved with multidisciplinary approaches using collaboration between different specialties such as psychologists, physiotherapists, nutritionists, rheumatologists.
- The focus on varied aspects of fibromyalgia such as physical, social, emotional will help in symptomatic management, and better outcomes.

FURTHER READING

1. Sarzi-Puttini P, Giorgi V, Marotto D, Atzeni F. Fibromyalgia: an update on clinical characteristics, aetiopathogenesis and treatment. Nat Rev Rheumatol 2020;16:645–60.
2. Di Carlo M, Bianchi B, Salaffi F, Pellegrino G, Iannuccelli C, Giorgi V, et al. Fibromyalgia: one year in review 2024. Clin Exp Rheumatol. 2024;42:1141–9.
3. Wasti AZ, Mackawy AMH, Hussain A, Huq M, Ahmed H, Memon AG. Fibromyalgia interventions, obstacles and prospects: narrative review. Acta Myol 2023;42:71–81.

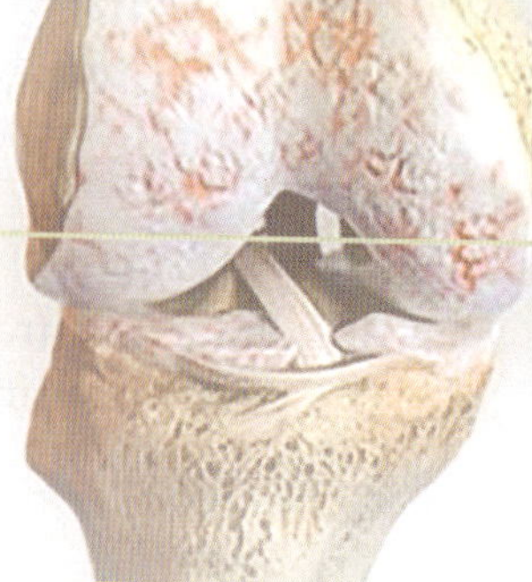

Chronic Fatigue Syndrome

N Kavya Devi

INTRODUCTION

Chronic fatigue syndrome (CFS), otherwise known as neurasthenia or myalgic encephalomyelitis (ME), is a complex biologic multisystem disease characterised not only by disabling fatigue but also by cognitive dysfunction, insomnia, dysautonomia and exercise intolerance leading to impairment of social, vocational, occupational and activities of daily living. Despite high prevalence and morbidity, CFS is undiagnosed/misdiagnosed in 91% of cases.

Occurrence of CFS is multi-factorial with complex interplay of genetics, environmental, infections, autoimmunity, physical and mental stress. CFS occurs most commonly in females (F:M 3:1), the typical age of onset often falls within two peak periods: late adolescence (10–19 years) and early middle age (30–39 years).

Clinical Features

Persistence of fatigue and post-expertional malaise for more than 50% of time and for at least 6 months without any underlying medical cause are the classical symptoms of CFS (Table 5.1).

Table 5.1: Clinical features of chronic fatigue syndrome	
Symptoms and signs	*Description*
Persistent fatigue	Sudden onset, not relieved by rest and worsens with activity
Post-exertional fatigue	Immediate or delayed onset of physical or cognitive fatigability to previously tolerated activities.
Unrefreshing sleep	Feeling unrested /unwell regardless of duration of sleep.
Cognitive impairment	Brain fog, decreased attention, memory and reaction time.
Orthostatic intolerance	Prolonged immobile upright position causes palpitations, syncope, light-headedness.
Autonomic dysfunction	Nausea, vomiting, drenching night sweats, dizziness, and intolerance to alcohol and other medications.
Influenza-like symptoms	Sore throat, tender lymph nodes

(Contd.)

(*Contd.*)

Symptoms and signs	Description
Gastrointestinal	Constipation, diarrhea, anorexia, bloating
Genitourinary	Increased urinary frequency/urgency and nocturia
Respiratory	Air hunger, thermoregulatory issues
Musculoskeletal	Polymyalgia, polyarthralgias

Diagnosis

As there are no specific diagnostic biomarkers, diagnosis depends entirely on clinical history and physical examination, ruling out all possible alternative causes (Table 5.2) and applying newer diagnostic criteria (Box 5.1)

Table 5.2: Alternative causes of fatigue

Causes of fatigue	Test ordered
Endocrine disorders	Thyroid profile Four-point salivary cortisol-to identify the abnormal diurnal cortisol patterns
Metabolic profile	Complete blood picture ESR, CRP RBS, CUE Liver function tests Renal function tests Serum electrolytes Creatine phosphokinase Serum calcium, magnesium, ferritin
Vitamin panel	Vitamin D, B_{12}
Infection panel	HIV, HBsAg, HCV Mantoux test, blood and urine cultures Treponemal tests Epstein-Barr virus, cytomegalovirus, parvovirus B19 panel
Autonomic dysfunction	10-minute NASA lean test or stand test Tilt table test
Sleep disorders	Overnight oximetry, polysomnography
Rheumatology disorders	ANA, rheumatoid factor
Cardiopulmonary tests	Chest X-ray, CT chest, ECG, 2D Echo, 24-hour Holter monitor, exercise test
Psychiatry screens	Questionnaire
Cancer screen	Age-appropriate screen tests

Box 5.1: The 2015 NAM diagnostic criteria for CFS

Diagnosis requires the following three symptoms
1. New or definite onset impairment in activities accompanied by fatigue for more than 6 months and is not substantially alleviated by rest,
2. Post-exertional malaise (PEM), and
3. Unrefreshing sleep

(*Contd.*)

(Contd.)

At least one of two following manifestations is also required
1. Cognitive impairment
2. Orthostatic intolerance
Symptoms should be of at least moderate intensity and present at least 50% of the time during a 6-month period

Treatment

There is no definite cure for CFS. Pharmacological and non-pharmacological measures are summarised in Table 5.3.

Symptom	*Non-pharmacological*	*Pharmacological*
Fatigue	Healthy diet Pacing therapy	Low dose naltrexone or aripiprazole, vitamin supplements.
Post-exertional malaise	Pace physical and cognitive activity. Assistive devices to conserve energy.	Low dose aripiprazole
Orthostatic intolerance	Salt, electrolyte and fluid loading. Compression stockings	Fludrocortisone, midodrine, pyridostigmine, low-dose beta blockers, alpha-adrenergic agonists ivabradine
Insomnia	Sleep hygiene practices. Meditation. Earplugs and eye masks. Blue light filters.	Hypnotics Low dose tricyclic Antidepressants Melatonin
Cognitive dysfunction and fatigue	Cognitive pacing simple memory aids	Methylphenidate, modafinil, caffeine if tolerated.
Pain	Pacing of activities. Hot or cold packs. Physiotherapy, massage, acupuncture. Meditation. Neurofeedback techniques.	NSAIDS Muscle relaxants Acetaminophen Opioids—Tramadol Serotonin—norepinephrine reuptake inhibitors
Gastrointestinal issues	Avoid caffeine, alcohol, spicy food, sugar, dairy.	Antidiarrheals Fibre and motility agents for constipation. Rifaximin, metronidazole for intestinal bacteria

Table 5.3: Management of CFS

Prognosis

CFS tends to have a more favorable prognosis when initial fatigue levels are low. Conversely, factors associated with a poor prognosis include older age, the presence of underlying psychiatric disorders, and a persistent belief in the severity of the illness.

Clinical Snippet

A 45-year-old lady X who was active in occupational and household tasks, presented with a 6 months history of exhaustion, myalgias, difficulty falling asleep, headache and decreased concentration. Frustrated with this, she restricted herself to home and had multiple speciality consultations with all tests being normal. Psychiatrist ruled out major depression as her fatigue is associated with more pains, unrefreshing sleep, worsening symptoms with exercise whereas depressive patients cop their fatigue with exercise, have less pains and anhedonia with fatigue. She had no tender points on examination unlike fibromyalgia. Finally, a diagnosis of chronic fatigue syndrome was made.

She was advised CBT, pacing therapy and stretching exercises. Started on amitriptyline 10 mg for improving mood and quality of sleep. As a result, she has been able to manage her daily activities more effectively.

FURTHER READING

1. US Institute of Medicine. Beyond Myalgic Encephalomyelitis/ Chronic Fatigue Syndrome: Redefining an Illness. Washington, DC: The National Academies Press; 2015.
2. Carruthers BM, van de Sande MI, De Meirleir KL, et al. Myalgic encephalomyelitis: International Consensus Criteria. J Intern Med. 2011 Oct;270(4):327–38.
3. Myalgic Encephalomyelitis/Chronic Fatigue Syndrome: Essentials of Diagnosis and Management. Bateman, Lucinda, et al. Mayo Clinic Proceedings, Volume 96, Issue 11,2861–78.

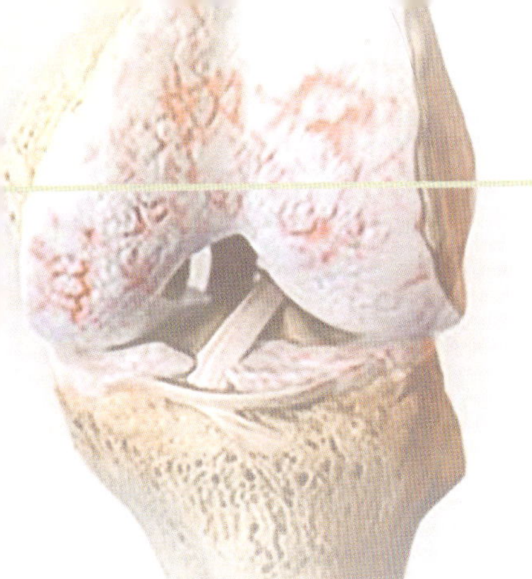

Laboratory Investigations

6. Approach to Lab Investigations in Rheumatology

Approach to Lab Investigations in Rheumatology

Kushagra Gupta, Vinod Ravindran

CONCEPT OF LAB INVESTIGATIONS IN RHEUMATOLOGY

Rheumatology is one of the trickiest subspecialties of medicine. This is primarily because there are no single objective tests for making a diagnosis of a rheumatic disease unlike other specialties. For example, in diabetes, if your HbA1c is more than 6.5, you have diabetes, there is no doubt about it! However, when we talk about rheumatoid arthritis, rheumatoid factor (RF) and anti-CCP positivity do not mean that the patient indeed has RA. This chapter reviews when and how to order and interpret lab tests in rheumatology.

When to order a test in Rheumatology?

Always consider pre-test probability for a test when suspecting an autoimmune condition (Fig. 6.1). Always ask yourself, what will I do if the test comes back positive? Will the diagnosis be confirmed after the test?

Let's take an example; a patient comes to you with a cavitary lung lesion. Considering the prevalence, a possibility of TB is most likely in our setting. But you order an autoimmune panel along with other tests. ANCA by ELISA (Anti-PR3) comes back positive, raising the possibility of vasculitis. Now what do you do? The pre-test probability for this patient to have vasculitis is not very high. ANCA false positivity has been reported in TB. Hence treating this patient with steroids only based on a positive ANCA would be a gamble.

Ordering tests with low pretest probability adds more confusion, loss in physician confidence and unnecessary drain of patient finances.

Approach for a Patient with Arthralgia

Diagnostic testing depends on the number and pattern of joints involved (Table 6.1)
- Presence of clinical symptoms (inflammatory pain) and signs (synovitis) is essential. Lab tests cannot confirm a diagnosis of arthritis in the absence of symptoms.
- False positives are common and vice versa is also true (Table 6.2).
- Synovial fluid examination can help differentiate between inflammatory and non-inflammatory joint effusions.
- Uric acid as a cause of joint pains is always overestimated. Mild pains and aches are never due to uric acid.

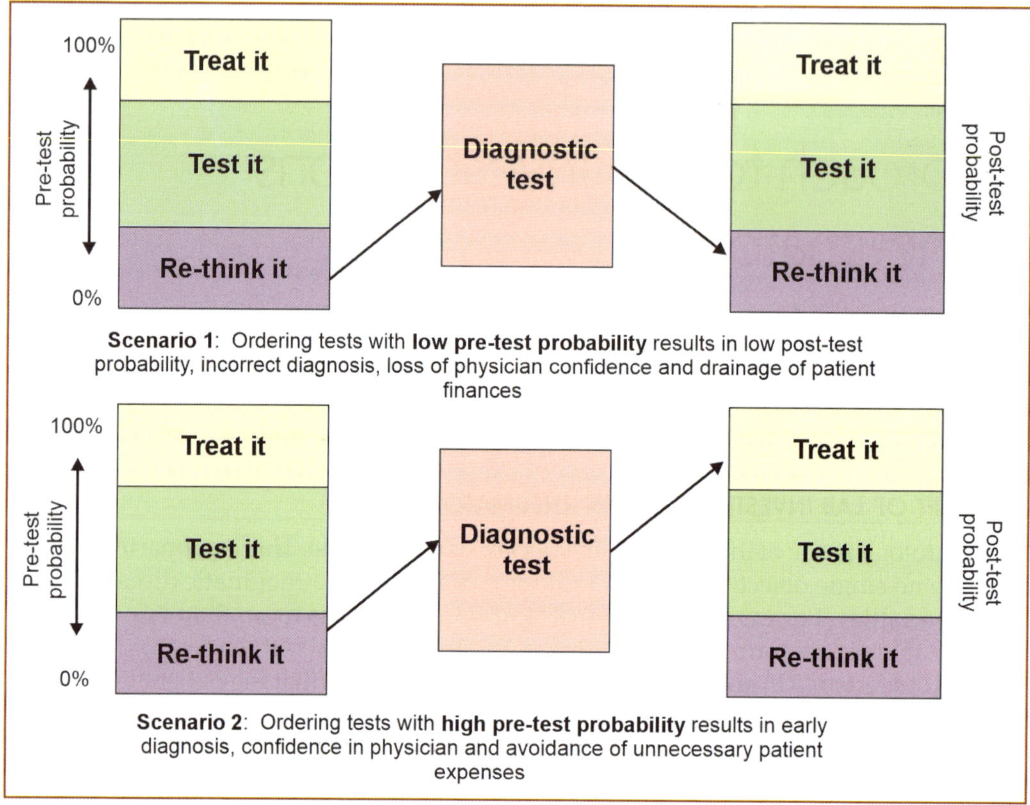

Fig. 6.1: Representation of clinical scenarios with low pre-test probability and high pre-test probability

Table 6.1: Suggested investigations based on clinical symptoms of a patient		
	Symptoms	*Suggested investigations and clues*
Joint Pain	Polyarthralgia	• Thyroid function • Diabetes screening • Vitamin D levels • Musculoskeletal USG (to rule out synovitis) • Fibromyalgia will be a diagnosis of exclusion
	Polyarthritis	• RF, Anti-CCP • ANA by IFA
	Oligoarthritis	• Synovial fluid analysis • RF, Anti-CCP • HLA-B27
	Monoarthritis	• Synovial fluid analysis • Uric acid • Musculoskeletal USG (identify hemarthrosis, double contour sign in gout, synovitis) • RF, anti-CCP (rarely there maybe monoarticular RA)

(Contd.)

(Contd.)

Symptoms		*Suggested investigations and clues*
Back pain	Inflammatory	• HLA-B27 • X-ray Lumbosacral spine, MRI SI joints–to look for sacroiliitis or syndesmophytes
Fever (pyrexia of unknown origin)	After ruling out infections	• ANA by IFA • ANCA–ANCA-associated vasculitis—only in the presence of corroborative symptoms • Serum Ferritin—adult-onset Still's disease • PET-CT—large vessel vasculitis
Ocular inflammation	Anterior uveitis	• HLA-B27 • Serum ace levels (rule out sarcoidosis)
	Posterior uveitis	• HLA-B51—Behcet's disease • ANA by IFA • ANCA by IFA and ELISA • Serum ACE levels
	Scleritis	• RF, anti-CCP • ANA by IFA • ANCA by IFA and ELISA
ILD	After recognition of pattern on HRCT Chest	RF, anti-CCP ANA by IFA (presence of Raynaud's phenomenon) • Homogenous/speckled/nucleolar—get ENA profile • Cytoplasmic pattern—get myositis profile
Recurrent abortions/ thrombosis (Young CVA/ CAD)	Anticardiolipin antibody—IgM and IgG Anti β2 glycoprotein antibody—IgM and IgG Lupus anticoagulant (Levels above 40 IU are considered significant on 2 occasions 12 weeks apart)	

Note: All investigations should be ordered and interpreted in the appropriate clinical context.
ACE: Angiotensin converting enzyme; ANA: Anti-nuclear antibody; ANCA: Anti-neutrophilic cytoplasmic antibody; Anti-CCP: Anti-cyclic citrullinated protein antibody; CTD: Connective tissue disease; HLA: Human leucocyte antigen; HRCT: High resolution computed tomography; ILD: Interstitial lung disease; IFA: Immunofluorescence; ENA: Extractable nuclear antigen; MRI: Magnetic resonance imaging; PET: Positron emission tomography; RF: Rheumatoid factor; USG: ultrasound

Table 6.2: Sensitivity and specificity of common lab tests for diagnosis of rheumatic diseases			
Lab Tests	*Sensitivity*	*Specificity*	*For disease*
ESR/CRP	50–60%	<40%	RA
RF	60%	85%	RA
Anti-CCP	65%	98%	RA
ANA	98%	57%	SLE
Uric acid	89%	61%	Gout
HLA-B27	80%	95%	Spondyloarthritis
c-ANCA	64%	95%	GPA
p-ANCA	58%	80–90%	MPA

GPA: Granulomatosis with polyangiitis; MPA: Microscopic polyangiitis

Interpreting ANA Test

Another common problem in rheumatology is the interpretation of the ANA test (Tables 6.2 and 6.3). Some key points to consider:
- ANA should always be obtained by immunofluorescence (IFA) and not ELISA.
- A titer of 1:80 and above is considered significant. 15% of the normal healthy population can have a positive ANA (1:80) .
- ANA patterns can be misleading and should not be interpreted without proper experience.
- ENA profile may be needed to characterise disease further
- p-ANCA can sometimes be falsely reported positive in patients with a positive ANA.

Clues to Multisystemic Diseases

When dealing with multisystemic diseases, it is not always possible to define a preset line of investigations to follow. However, some clues can help you stay on top of things.
- Leucocytosis does not always mean sepsis. It can due to systemic vasculitides and autoinflammatory conditions (like adult onset Still's disease, etc.).
- ESR>100 in a stable patient is usually seen in either malignancy or autoimmune conditions.
- A low serum albumin means that there is a chronic undifferentiated inflammatory pathology at play that needs further workup.
- Low ESR and CRP can often be misleading.
- High globulins (polyclonal on protein electrophoresis) hint towards a diagnosis of rheumatic diseases.
- Urine analysis is the most underrated investigation. It can often provide you with clues about your diagnosis.
- In case of persistent transaminitis, always rule out the possibility of hemolysis and myositis.

Table 6.3: Interpretation of connective tissue diseases based on ENA testing		
ANA pattern	*Antigens*	*Etiologies*
Any 'Nuclear pattern' (Homogenous, speckled, centromere, nucleolar, etc.) in titres above 1:80	Ro52 Ro60 La	Sjögren syndrome
	SCL70 or centromere antibodies	Scleroderma
	U1RNP (high titres, 3+)	MCTD
	Ro52, Ro60, U1RNP, Sm, dsDNA and some other antibodies (also known as full house pattern)	SLE
	DFS70	No autoimmune disease in patient
	All other antibodies (either alone or in combination) are not specific for any particular disease	
'Cytoplasmic pattern' on ANA	Could be suggestive of underlying myositis or progressive ILD false positives are also common	

Conclusion

In the last decade, there has been an exponential increase in the number of lab tests available for rheumatic diseases. It is important to remember that no test can be used standalone for making a diagnosis. Pattern recognition and timely referral to a rheumatologist is the key to making a diagnosis.

FURTHER READING

1. Bossuyt X, De Langhe E, Borghi MO, Meroni PL. Understanding and interpreting antinuclear antibody tests in systemic rheumatic diseases. Nat Rev Rheumatol. 2020 Dec;16(12):715–726.
2. Allard-Chamard H, Boire G. Serologic Diagnosis of Rheumatoid Arthritis. Clin Lab Med. 2019 Dec;39(4):525–537.

Section

III

Autoimmune and Inflammatory Diseases

Rheumatoid Arthritis

Keerthi Talari Bommakanti

INTRODUCTION

Rheumatoid arthritis (RA) is a chronic autoimmune disease with about 60% heritability, involving HLA-DRB1 alleles, citrullination of peptides, and environmental triggers like smoking.

Clinical Features

RA typically presents as symmetric, polyarticular arthritis, affecting the small joints of the hands (MCP and PIP) and feet (MTP), while sparing the DIP and 1st CMC joints. Larger joints can also be involved. Atlanto-axial joint involvement may cause neck pain, instability, and in severe cases, spinal cord compression.

Deformities

Deformity	Description
Swan-neck	Hyperextension of PIP and flexion of DIP joints.
Boutonnière	Flexion of PIP and hyperextension of DIP joints.
Piano key sign	Increased mobility of the ulnar styloid from synovitis and instability in the inferior radioulnar joint.
Dorsal Subluxation	Dorsal displacement of carpal bones causing wrist deformity.

Others: Ulnar deviation at MCPs

Extra-articular Manifestations

RA is a systemic disease that can affect various organs and tissues beyond the joints:

- **Rheumatoid nodules:** Firm, subcutaneous nodules typically found on pressure points and extensor aspects such as the elbows and fingers.
- **Pulmonary involvement:** Interstitial lung disease, pleuritis, and pulmonary nodules are common pulmonary manifestations.
- **Cardiovascular involvement:** Increased risk of atherosclerosis, pericarditis, and myocarditis.
- **Ocular involvement:** Keratoconjunctivitis sicca (dry eyes), scleritis, and episcleritis.
- **Hematologic involvement:** Anemia of chronic disease, thrombocytosis, and Felty's syndrome (RA, splenomegaly, and neutropenia).

Classification Criteria

The 1987 ACR criteria for RA often missed early cases, leading to delayed diagnosis before joint erosions developed. The 2010 RA classification criteria, developed by ACR and the EULAR, help in classifying RA before the development of erosive joint disease. Classification criteria are mainly meant to have a homogenous population for research purposes.

These criteria apply to patients with definite synovitis not better explained by another diagnosis. A total score of 6 out of 10 is needed for a classification of RA:

Criterion	Score
Joint involvement	
1 large joint	0
2–10 large joints	1
1–3 small joints	2
4–10 small joints	3
>10 joints (at least 1 small joint)	5
Serology	
Negative RF and negative ACPA	0
Low-positive RF or low-positive ACPA	2
High-positive RF or high-positive ACPA	3
Acute-phase reactants	
Normal CRP and normal ESR	0
Abnormal CRP or abnormal ESR	1
Duration of symptoms	
<6 weeks	0
≥6 weeks	1

Diagnosis

RA diagnosis is based on clinical evaluation, laboratory tests, and imaging.

- **Serology:**
  - *Rheumatoid factor (RF):* Positive in about 70–80% of patients with RA.
  - *Anti-citrullinated protein antibody (ACPA):* Highly specific for RA, present in 60–70% of patients.

  Both RF and ACPA need not be repeated once positive unless the reliability of the test is in doubt.
- **Acute-phase reactants:**
  - *C-reactive protein (CRP):* Elevated in active disease.
  - *Erythrocyte sedimentation rate (ESR):* Elevated in active disease.
- **Imaging:**
  - *X-rays:* Show joint space narrowing, erosions, and periarticular osteopenia.
  - *Ultrasound and MRI:* Useful for detecting early joint inflammation and erosions not visible on X-rays.

Disease Activity Measures

Disease activity in RA is assessed using composite indices like the Disease Activity Score in 28 joints (DAS28), Clinical Disease Activity Index (CDAI), Simplified Disease Activity Index (SDAI), and patient-reported outcomes. DAS28 includes joint counts, erythrocyte sedimentation rate (ESR)/C-reactive protein (CRP), and patient assessment, with scores indicating remission (<2.6) to high activity (>5.1). CDAI uses joint counts and both patient and physician assessments, ranging from remission ($\leq$2.8) to high activity (>22). SDAI adds CRP, with remission at $\leq$3.3 and high activity >26. Patient-reported tools like the Health Assessment Questionnaire (HAQ) and Routine Assessment of Patient Index Data 3 (RAPID3) assess function, pain, and health. These measures guide treatment, targeting remission or low disease activity to improve long-term outcomes.

Treatment

Early diagnosis and prompt initiation of disease-modifying antirheumatic drugs (DMARDs) within 12 weeks improves rheumatoid arthritis outcomes, following a treat-to-target (T2T) approach for remission or low disease activity. Glucocorticoids provide rapid inflammation control and serve as bridging therapy before DMARDs act, while NSAIDs offer pain relief but are not disease-modifying.

Disease-Modifying Antirheumatic Drug (DMARD) Therapy

Conventional Synthetic DMARDs

Drug Name	Dose	Toxicity	Special Notes
Methotrexate	7.5 mg to 25 mg weekly	Hepatotoxicity, bone marrow suppression, GI intolerance	Folic acid supplementation recommended
Sulfasalazine	2–3 g daily in two divided doses	GI intolerance, rash, hepatitis, DRESS	Usually safe if tolerated for 3 months
Leflunomide	20 mg daily	Hepatotoxicity, loose stools, teratogenicity	Long half-life, to be avoided in reproductive age group
Hydroxy-chloroquine	200–400 mg daily	Retinal toxicity, slate grey skin pigmentation	Baseline and annual eye exams
Iguratimod	25 mg twice daily	Hepatotoxicity, GI disturbances	Used primarily in Asian countries

Biologic DMARDs

All biologic agents are started only after certain screening tests which usually include viral serologies, chest X-ray and latent TB screening.

Drug Name	Dose	Toxicity/Contraindications	Special Notes
Adalimumab	40 mg every other week	Infection risk	TNF inhibitor
Etanercept	50 mg weekly	Infection risk	TNF inhibitor
Infliximab	3–5 mg/kg every 8 weeks	Infection risk, infusion reactions	TNF inhibitor
Rituximab	1000 mg twice, two weeks apart	Infusion reactions, infection risk	B cell depleting agent
Tocilizumab	4-8 mg/kg every 4 weeks	Infection risk, GI perforation	IL-6 receptor inhibitor, requires monitoring for lipid abnormalities

Other biologics approved for RA, but currently not available in India are not discussed.

Targeted Synthetic DMARDs

Drug Name	Dose	Toxicity/Contraindications	Special Notes
Tofacitinib	5 mg twice daily or 11 mg XR once daily	Infection risk especially zoster, deep vein thrombosis	Janus kinase inhibitor suitable for monotherapy
Baricitinib	2 mg once daily	Major adverse cardiovascular events, Weight gain, lipid abnormalities	
Upadacitinib	15 mg once daily		

Prognosis

The prognosis of rheumatoid arthritis (RA) has improved with early diagnosis and DMARDs, enabling remission or low disease activity. Without proper treatment, RA can cause joint destruction, disability, and increased cardiovascular risk. Early, aggressive treatment and regular monitoring are crucial for preventing progression and ensuring better long-term outcomes.

Clinical Snippet

- A 45-year-old woman with 3-year history of joint pain and swelling, primarily in wrists and hands, with morning stiffness and joint deformities.
- **Physical exam:** Synovitis in MCP and PIP joints, ulnar deviation, boutonnière deformity, rheumatoid nodules.
- **Investigations:** Positive RF, anti-CCP, elevated ESR (40 mm/hr) and CRP (25 mg/L), X-rays show joint erosions.
- **Management:**
  - Methotrexate 10–15 mg weekly, folic acid 1 mg daily.
  - Consider low-dose glucocorticoids as bridging therapy.
  - Monitor disease activity every 3 months
  - Taper glucocorticoids, optimize DMARDs on follow up

FURTHER READING

1. Hochberg MC, Silman AJ, Smolen JS, Weinblatt ME, Weisman MH, editors. *Rheumatology*. 8th ed. Philadelphia: Elsevier; 2019. p. 749–874.

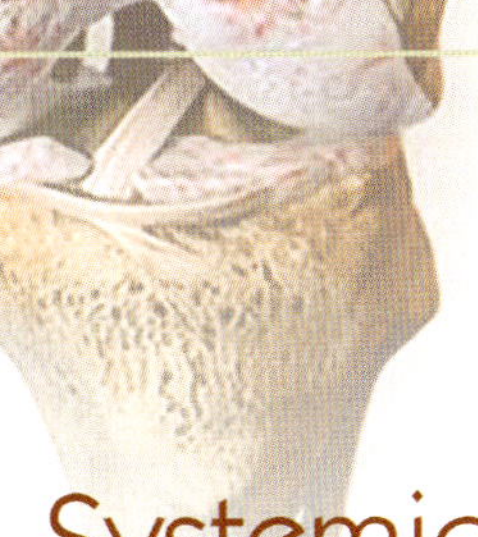

Systemic Lupus Erythematosus (SLE)

Irlapati Rajendra Vara Prasad

INTRODUCTION

Lupus is considered as a prototype multisystem autoimmune disease with characteristic flares and remissions throughout the disease course. It commonly affects skin, muscles and joints of young women, but can involve all major organ systems if untreated.

It is common in India with an estimated point prevalence of 3.2/100,000 population according to a 1993 study, which could be more now.

Disease is triggered by unknown environmental factors in a genetically predisposed individual. The inflammation is primarily driven by antinuclear antibodies and Type 1 interferons.

Clinical Features

The clinical features include constitutional features and symptoms related to organ involvement.

Clinical domains	Clinical features
Mucocutaneous manifestations (10–50%)	Acute, subacute and chronic cutaneous lesions. Acute lesions correlate with disease activity
Arthritis (90%)	Non-erosive arthritis
Hematological manifestations (85%)	Autoimmune hemolytic anemia (14%), thrombocytopenia (30%), leucopenia (20–40%), macrophage activation syndrome (5%)
Cardiac manifestations (50%)	Pericarditis (25%), myocarditis, valve regurgitation, nonbacterial thrombotic endocarditis, pulmonary arterial hypertension
Pulmonary manifestations (50%)	Pleural effusion, pneumonia, ILD, diffuse alveolar hemorrhage and shrinking lung syndrome
Renal (30–50%)	Lupus nephritis (associated with anti-double-stranded DNA-antibodies and decreased complement levels)
Neuropsychiatric manifestations (60%)	Headache, mood disorders, cognitive impairment, seizures, psychosis, polyneuropathy and stroke
Gastrointestinal manifestations (40%)	Ascitis, hepatitis, mesenteric vasculitis, proteinlosing enteropathy, pancreatitis and intestinal pseudo-obstruction

Diagnosis

Diagnosis of lupus can be made from detailed clinical history taking, meticulous clinical examination supported by serological tests like antinuclear antibodies and anti-double stranded DNA antibodies. Systemic Lupus International Collaborating Clinics (SLICC) criteria (specificity 97%, sensitivity 84%) are used for classifying an individual patient.

The following tests can help in diagnosing and assessing activity and damage of SLE.

Test	Abnormalities
Complete blood counts	Cytopenias
Liver function tests	Elevated liver enzymes Low albumin-nephrotic syndrome, protein losing enteropathy
Renal function tests	Azotemia–Nephritis Hypokalemia–Distal RTA, steroid related
Complete urine examination	Active sediment and pyuria-nephritis
CPK	Myositis
LDH	Hemolysis
Serological tests	
Anti-ds DNA (70%)	Diagnosis (97% specific) and disease activity (vasculitis, nephritis)
Anti-Smith (25%)	Diagnosis (98% specific) and disease activity
Antiphospholipid antibodies (30–50%)	Thrombocytopenia,risk for thrombosis and adverse pregnancy outcomes
Complement C3 and C4 levels	Low in active disease
Anti-Ro/SS-A (30%) & Anti-LA/SS-B (10%)	Neonatal lupus, subacute cutaneous lupus, Sjögren's syndrome overlap
Anti-ribosomal P (20%)	CNS lupus
Antihistone (70%)	Drug-induced lupus
Anti-RNP (40%)	Overlap features of several rheumatic syndromes including SLE
Antierythrocyte (60%)	Measured as direct Coombs test

Treatment

The goal of the treatment is to achieve remission or low disease activity, reduce disease flares, organ damage accrual, minimize or avoid use of steroids and improve quality of life. Treatment is to be tailored to the disease severity guided by disease activity assessment, comorbidities and patient preferences.

Drug	Indications	Important adverse effects	
Hydroxychloroquine (Antimalarial) mg/Kg	Reduces disease flares. Useful for arthritis and cutaneous manifestations	Retinopathy, gastritis, skin pigment abnormalities	

(Contd.)

(Contd.)

Drug	Indications	Important adverse effects	
Glucocorticoids 1 mg–1000 mg	Active disease	Infection, weight gain, hypertension, hyperglycemia, mood or sleep disturbance, peptic ulcers, osteoporosis, osteonecrosis, myopathy, impaired wound healing, adrenal suppression	
Azathioprine (Purine inhibitor) (1–2 mg/kg)	Maintenance therapy for nephritis and steroid sparing agent	Hepatitis, leucopenia, rarely malignancies	
Cyclophosphamide (Alkylating agent) 500–1000 mg/m^2	Severe organ threatening disease, Induction therapy for nephritis and neuropsychiatric manifestations	Marrow suppression, ovarian toxicity, hemorrhagic cystitis and rarely malignancy	Classically used in bi weekly (ELNT regimen) or monthly (NIH regimen)pulses
Methotrexate (Folate antimetabolite) 10–25 mg/week	Moderate disease, especially for cutaneous and articular symptoms	Gastrointestinal, hepatotoxicity, headache, infection; alopecia, mucositis; interstitial pneumonitis	
Mycophenolate mofetil/mycophenolic acid (purine synthesis inhibitor) 2–3 gm in two divided doses	Moderate to severe disease. Induction and maintenance for lupus nephritis, and steroid sparing agent	Gastrointestinal, cytopenias, infections	
Tacrolimus (Calcineurin inhibitor) 3–5 mg/day in two divided doses	Moderate to severe disease. lupus nephritis, steroid sparing agent	Nephrotoxicity, hypertension, infections	Used in multitargeted therapy for nephritis, safe in pregnancy
Cyclosporine (Calcineurin inhibitor) 2–5 mg/kg	Moderate to severe disease. lupus nephritis, steroid sparing agent	Nephrotoxicity, hypertension, infections	Used in multitargeted therapy for nephritis, safe in pregnancy
Voclosporin (Calcineurin inhibitor) 23.7 mg twice daily	Moderate to severe disease; LN therapy	Nephrotoxicity, hypertension, infections	
Rituximab 1 g IV given twice 2 wk apart or 375 mg/m2 IV weekly for 4 doses B-cell Inhibition	Moderate to severe disease; can be considered for LN in combination with standard therapy	Infusion reaction, hypogammaglobulinemia, infections	

(Contd.)

(Contd.)

Drug	Indications	Important adverse effects	
Anifrolumab (type I interferon receptor Inhibitor) 300 mg IV every 4 wk	Moderate to severe disease; primarily effective for skin disease	Infusion reaction, skin and respiratory infections	Not and CNS involvement
Belimumab (10 mg/kg IV every 4 wk or 200 mg subcutaneously weekly) B cell inhibitor	Moderate to severe disease; LN therapy in conjunction with standard therapy	Infusion reactions, infections, depression	Not for active nephritis and CNS involvement

Prognosis

Prognosis of lupus patients is steadily improving with recent therapeutic advances and disease awareness. Need to be on regular medication to control disease activity and prevent disease flares. Permanent complete remissions (absence of symptoms with no treatment) occur in <5%. Mortality is high in the initial part of the disease due to infections and to some extent active disease, whereas cardiovascular disease is higher later in life. ESRD is seen in 10% of lupus nephritis patients.

Clinical Snippet

A young girl, age 16 years came with intermittent fever for the past 6 months associated with fatigue and loss of appetite. Subsequently she, photosensitivity and excessive hair loss. Over the next one month, she developed retrosternal chest pain, pedal edema progressing into anasarca.

She was treated for enteric fever based on clinical suspicion in the first month of her symptoms. After 3 months she was found to have pleural effusions on chest radiograph for which she was initiated on empirical anti-tuberculous treatment with no relief. On noticing clinical deterioration this patient was referred to a tertiary hospital.

On clinical evaluation, the patient had puffy face, pedal edema, sparse hair, faint malar rash, palatal erosion, cervical lymphadenopathy. She had hypertension and signs of pleural and pericardial effusion.

Lab evaluation showed mild leucopenia, elevated ESR, mild transaminitis, normal creatinine, active urinary sediment with proteinuria of 2 gm/day, low C3 and C4 levels, with elevated dsDNA antibody titres. Her renal biopsy was suggestive of Class IV lupus nephritis. Antiphospholipid antibodies were not present.

She was started on IV methylprednisolone 500 mg/day for 3 days followed by 0.5 mg/kg BW oral steroids, along with cyclophosphamide pulse therapy, hydroxychloroquine and supportive treatment. After 6 months the patient is in clinical and laboratory remission without steroids and on maintenance immunosuppression with mycophenolate mofetil.

FURTHER READING

1. Siegel CH, Sammaritano LR. Systemic Lupus Erythematosus: A Review. JAMA. 2024 Apr 8.
2. Kehl A, Wallace DJ. Overview and clinical presentation. InDubois' Lupus Erythematosus and Related Syndromes 2024 Oct 1 (pp. 413–420).
3. Hahn, Bevra Hannahs, and Maureen McMahon. "Systemic Lupus Erythematosus." *Harrison's Principles of Internal Medicine, 21e* Eds. Joseph Loscalzo, et al. McGraw-Hill Education, 2022.

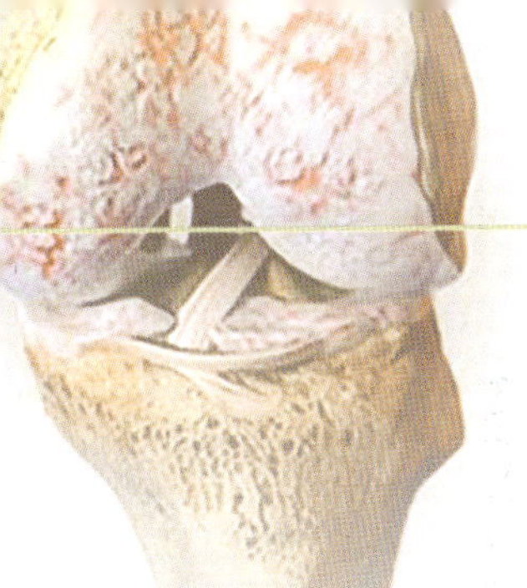

Antiphospholipid Syndrome

Ranjan Gupta

INTRODUCTION

Antiphospholipid syndrome (APS) is an autoimmune disease characterized clinically by intravascular thrombosis or pregnancy morbidity and serologically by the presence of persistent antiphospholipid antibodies (APLA) (including anti-cardiolipin antibodies [ACLA] or anti-β2-glycoprotein-I antibodies [anti-β2GPI] immunoglobulin IgG or IgM), abnormal coagulation assay (presence of inhibitor of phospholipid-dependent clotting—the lupus anti-coagulant [LAC] test), or both. It can exist as an isolated disease or in association with other rheumatic diseases, the commonest being systemic lupus erythematosus (SLE). The morbidity in APS is related to mainly 2 domains namely vascular morbidity which manifests as vessel thrombosis causing ischemia leading to organ damage and pregnancy morbidity in the form of recurrent pregnancy losses (RPL). However, its manifestations may range from being asymptomatic to catastrophic APS (CAPS).

The pathogenesis of APS is characterized by shifting of the phosphatidylserine to the outer layer of the cell membrane of the apoptotic cells, endothelial cells and trophoblasts which are bound by the β2GpI molecules which are in turn are bound by the APLs leading to generation of C5a via activation of classic complement pathway. This causes activation of monocytes and polymorphonuclear cells that cause tissue damage by their cytokine release.

Diagnosis

The original Sapporo classification criteria for APS developed in 1999 were revised in 2006 but did not include manifestations like livedo reticularis, thrombocytopenia, autoimmune hemolytic anemia. The recently revised 2023 ACR/EULAR classification criteria have included these minor manifestations as well as the grade of positivity of APLs. For diagnosis of APS, persistent positivity (at 12 weeks) of APLs is mandatory in both these criteria because transient positivity for autoantibodies can occur during acute illnesses and infections.

Risk Stratification in APS

First step in the management of APS includes risk stratification based on the APLA profile.

1. Patients with isolated APL antibody positivity in low-medium titres is considered as low risk profile.
2. Medium-high titres are considered as medium risk profile.
3. Persistent positive high titres of APLA, LAC positivity, triple antibody positivity and double antibody positivity is considered to be high risk APLA profile.

Treatment

Vascular APS

Primary thromboprophylaxis (i.e. patients who have never had a vascular thrombosis) with low dose aspirin (75–100 mg/day) is recommended in:
1. Asymptomatic carriers with high risk profile patients with or without underlying rheumatic diseases and
2. In patients with past history of obstetric APS even with a low risk profile.

For secondary thromboprophylaxis (i.e. patients who have had a vascular thrombosis while being APLA positive):
1. A moderate intensity anticoagulation is recommended keeping international normalized (INR) ratio between 2 and 3.
2. For patients who develop a vascular thrombosis while on moderate-intensity anticoagulation, a higher intensity of anticoagulation, i.e. INR between 3 and 4 is recommended.
3. Other options for such patients are adding aspirin to anticoagulation and shifting to low molecular weight heparin.
4. The duration of anticoagulation is recommended to be lifelong.

It is important to note that direct oral anticoagulants (DOACs) like rivaroxaban, etc. are not recommended for routine use in APS and vitamin K antagonists (VKAs) like warfarin is the first drug of choice for this. DOACs are only conditionally recommended for use in patients who are already on DOACs with a stable anticoagulation, patients unwilling for INR monitoring and patients with serious adverse effects or contraindications for use of VKAs.

Obstetric APS

1. All patients with obstetric APS should receive LDA if otherwise not contraindicated.
2. Patients who have RPL while being on LDA, should be treated with a prophylactic dose of LMWH starting as soon as pregnancy is confirmed till the end of puerperium period.
3. If RPLs still continue, LMWH should be initiated before conception itself.
4. Pregnant ladies with vascular APS with/without obstetric APS should be treated with therapeutic doses of LMWH as mentioned above.

Other Manifestations in APS

1. These manifestations like AIHA, thrombocytopenia, etc. should be managed as per the principles of their management in other rheumatic diseases.
2. Treatment with immunomodulator medications routinely is not recommended in patients with APS for decreasing the titres of APLAs.

Catastrophic APS

This is the most severe and life-threatening manifestation of APS and is classified based on the criteria requiring documentation of thrombosis in three or more organs/tissues. It frequently presents as multi-organ failure syndrome. Timely diagnosis is important not just to prevent mortality but because the treatment includes anti-coagulation, steroids, plasma exchange, and in refractory cases, cyclophosphamide/rituximab.

FURTHER READING

1. Barbhaiya M, et al. Development of a new international antiphospholipid syndrome classification criteria phase I/II report: generation and reduction of candidate criteria. Arthritis Care Res (Hoboken) 2021;73(10):1490–1501.
2. Tektonidou MG, et al. EULAR recommendations for the management of antiphospholipid syndrome in adults. Ann Rheum Dis. 2019;78(10):1296–1304.
3. Asherson RA, et al. Catastrophic antiphospholipid syndrome: international consensus statement on classification criteria and treatment guidelines, Lupus 2003;12(7):530–534.

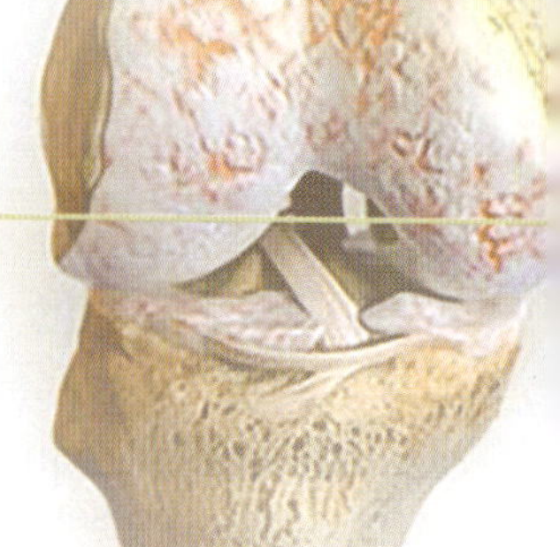

Spondyloarthritis

Muppalla Mowlika, Adapa Ramakrishnam Naidu

INTRODUCTION

Spondyloarthritis (SpA) is a group of autoimmune disorders characterised by axial, peripheral and extra-musculoskeletal manifestations. The axial involvement manifests as sacroiliitis, spondylitis and peripheral involvement in the form of arthritis, enthesitis and dactylitis. The extra-musculoskeletal manifestations include uveitis, inflammatory bowel disease, psoriasis and rarely aortitis, interstitial lung disease, IgA nephropathy and renal amyloidosis. SpA affects about 0.2 to 1.6% of the population worldwide. It is classified into axial and peripheral SpA. Axial SpA, a prototypic disease of SpA, is further classified into radiographic (r-axSpA) and non-radiographic SpA (nr-axSpA). The etiology of SpA is driven by genetic factors like HLA-B27 and non-HLA genes like ERAP 1, IL 17A and IL-23 polymorphisms and variable degrees of gut dysbiosis.

Clinical Features

The disease usually starts in third decade of life with male to female ratio of 2:1 in r-axSpA and 1:1 in nr-axSpA. The predominant manifestation of axSpA is inflammatory back pain, characterised by chronic low back pain, lasting more than three months with alternating buttock pain, worse in second part of night associated with nocturnal awakening, early morning stiffness, relieves with exercises and nonsteroidal anti-inflammatory drugs (NSAIDs).

Other manifestations are peripheral arthritis, defined as arthritis in limb joints except hips and shoulders occurs in about 25% of axSpA patients, and is usually asymmetrical mono/oligoarthritis with predominant lower limb involvement.

Hip arthritis occurs in 50% of cases, associated with poor prognosis. Shoulder arthritis occurs in 30% of cases, occurs late in the disease course.

Enthesitis is inflammation of the bony origin and insertion of ligaments, tendons, joint capsule, or fascia. It occurs in 30% of cases, more commonly at sites which are subjected to great physical stress like Achilles tendinitis and plantar fasciitis. It manifests as pain, stiffness with or without swellings. Enthesitis at costovertebral, costosternal, and manubriosternal joints causes chest pain, especially on sneezing and coughing.

Dactylitis is characterised by diffuse swelling of one or more fingers or toes, also known as sausage digit. It occurs due to the combination of synovitis, tenosynovitis, and enthesitis of the fingers and/or toes.

The extra-musculoskeletal manifestations include uveitis, psoriasis and inflammatory bowel disease. Acute anterior uveitis occurs in about 14 to 26% of axSpA cases and is typically sudden in onset, unilateral, alternating, recurring and manifests as painful red eye with photophobia, blurred vision and increased lacrimation. Posterior uveitis can be seen rarely with coexistent IBD.

Inflammatory bowel disease, includes Crohn's disease and ulcerative colitis. Up to 60% of axSpA patients have microscopic inflammatory gut lesions. Clinically apparent IBD with chronic diarrhea, pain abdomen and rectal bleeding is seen in about 7% of axSpA.

Prevalence of psoriasis in axSpA is seen in about 10% of cases, characterised by predominant peripheral joint involvement and worse prognosis.

Other rare extra-articular manifestations of the disease include aortitis, conduction abnormalities, restrictive lung disease, IgA nephropathy, renal amyloidosis, osteoporosis and increased vertebral fractures.

Diagnosis

HLA-B27 is positive in around 70 to 90% of patients with axSpA, but it can be positive in around 6 to 8% of general population. Elevation in acute phase reactants (ESR and CRP) can be seen in 40% of the patients.

Imaging includes X-ray and MRI of sacroiliac joints and spine. The presence of sacroiliitis on X-ray can be identified using modified New York criteria in patients with r-axSpA. Absence of X-ray changes with MRI evidence of sacroiliitis is known as nr-axSpA.

The current classification criteria in use to categorise axSpA-ASAS 2009 criteria

Table 10.1: Back pain ≥3 months and age at onset <45 years	
Sacroiliitis on imaging + ≥1 SpA features	*HLA B27 + ≥2 other SpA features*
Sacroiliitis on imaging Active inflammation on MRI highly suggestive of sacroiliitis associated with SpA. Or Definite radiographic sacroiliitis according to modified New York criteria	**SpA features** Inflammatory back pain Arthritis Enthesitis Uveitis Dactylitis Psoriasis Crohn disease or ulcerative colitis Good response to NSAIDs Family history of SpA HLA-B27 Elevated CRP

Peripheral SpA-ASAS 2011 criteria

Table 10.2: Arthritis or enthesitis or dactylitis	
Plus ≥1 of the following	Plus ≥1 of the following
Psoriasis	Arthritis
IBD	Enthesitis
Preceding infection	Dactylitis
HLA-B27	Inflammatory back pain in the past
Uveitis	Positive family history of SpA
Sacroiliitis on imaging	

Treatment

Non-pharmacological therapy includes physical therapy, smoking cessation.

Table 10.3: Pharmacological therapy				
Drug name	*Mode of action*	*Dose*	*Toxicity/ Contraindications*	*Special notes*
Celecoxib Etoricoxib	COX-2 inhibitor	100 mg BD 90 mg OD	Increased MACE events, renal adverse effects like papillary necrosis, AKI, interstitial nephritis. Less incidence of GI side effects compared to traditional NSAIDs	Initial choice of therapy for symptomatic relief, but doubtful role in reducing the rate of radiographic progression. The adverse effects often limits the long term use of NSAIDs.
Naproxen	COX-1 & COX-2 inhibitor	500 mg BD	GI side effects like nausea, peptic ulcers, GI bleeds, cardiovascular and renal side effects	
Sulfasalazine	Anti-inflammatory effects of 5ASA and sulfapyridine	2–3 gm/day	GI side effects like nausea, vomiting, diarrhoea, anaphylactic rash, hepatotoxicity, rarely agranulocytosis	For peripheral disease, not recommended in axial disease
Infliximab	TNF inhibitor	5 mg/kg IV at week 0, 2, 6, then every 8 weeks	Infusion and injection site reactions, increased risk of infections, rarely demyelination, malignancies	TNF inhibitors are initial bDMARDs of choice. Beneficial in axial and peripheral SpA
Adalimumab	TNF inhibitor	40 mg SC every 2 weeks		
Etanercept	TNF inhibitor	50 mg SC every weekly		Contraindicated in uveitis and IBD
Golimumab	TNF inhibitor	50 mg SC every 4 weeks		
Secukinumab	IL-17A inhibitor	150 mg SC at weeks 0, 1, 2, 3, 4, then every 4 weeks	Increased risk of fungal infections	Contraindicated in IBD
Tofacitinib	JAK-1 & JAK-2 inhibitor	5 mg BD	Increased risk of infections, MACE events, dyslipidemias	Considered in patients with inadequate response to TNF and IL-17 inhibitors.

Prognosis

SpA has a very unpredictable course. Radiographic damage may progress more quickly in men with r-axSpA. Life expectancy is reduced, particularly after 10 years of disease.

Functional limitation increases with disease duration. Overall, the first 10 years of disease are particularly important with respect to subsequent outcome. Most of the functional disability occurs within this period and is associated with the presence of peripheral arthritis, spinal radiographic changes, and development of bamboo spine. Anti-TNF therapy early in the disease course associated with less risk of radiographic progression. Causes of death include complications of the disease such as amyloidosis and spinal fractures, as well as cardiovascular, gastrointestinal, and renal disease.

Clinical Snippet

A 32-year-old male, presented with gradually progressive inflammatory low back pain from 3 years. Back pain improved temporarily with NSAIDs. On examination he had positive Patrick's and Schober's test. HLA-B27 was positive. ESR was 57mm/1st hour and CRP was 14 mg/dl. Imaging of X-ray sacroiliac joints showed irregularities and narrowing of bilateral sacroiliac joints, coinciding with grade 3 sacroilitis (modified New York criteria) and MR imaging had evidence of bilateral active sacroiliitis. He was initiated on TNF inhibitor therapy with Adalimumab subcutaneous once every two weeks. After receiving three to four doses of adalimumab he had significant improvement in his symptoms.

FURTHER READING

1. Sieper J, Poddubnyy D. Axial spondyloarthritis. The Lancet. 2017 Jul 1;390(10089):73–84.
2. Ramiro S, Nikiphorou E, Sepriano A et al. ASAS-EULAR recommendations for the management of axial spondyloarthritis: 2022 update. Annals of the rheumatic diseases. 2023 Jan 1;82(1):19–34.

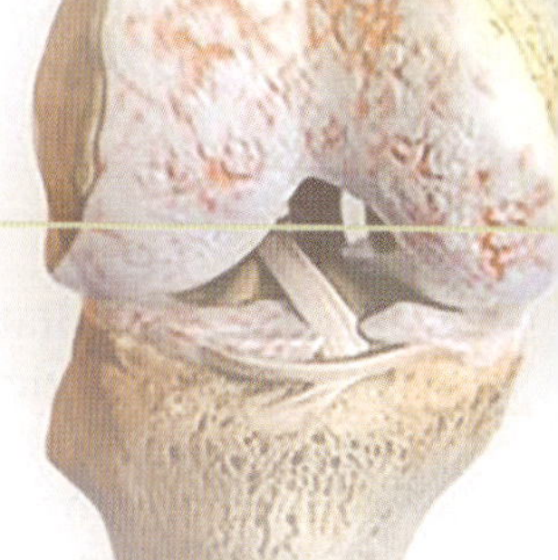

Reactive Arthritis

Srujana Arekal

INTRODUCTION

Reactive arthritis (ReA), also known as Reiter syndrome, is a type of spondyloarthropathy characterized by a combination of articular, entheseal, mucocutaneous, and ocular manifestations. These symptoms typically occur following genitourologic, enteric, or respiratory infections, and the causative organism cannot be cultured from synovial specimens.

Reactive arthritis (ReA) typically occurs in individuals aged 18 to 40, with peak incidence between 20 and 29 years. The risk is similar for men and women following enteric infections, however it is more common in men than women (9:1) after genitourinary infections.

Genetic factors such as the presence of HLA-B27, can increase both the risk and severity of the disease by 50%. HLA-B27 is implicated in the pathogenesis through molecular mimicry. Additionally, immune system abnormalities can contribute to these issues. Without appropriate management, the condition may progress to chronic, destructive arthritis. Development of reactive arthritis depends on four major factors (Fig. 11.1 and Table 11.1): Infection history, the role of cytokines, presence of HLA-B27 positivity, and gut microbiota.

PCR and immunocytochemical staining revealed bacterial triggers (lipopolysaccharides, or bacterial products) in synovial tissue, contributing to chronic arthritis. Reactive arthritis occurs in 3 to 10% of cases after exposure to potential agents.

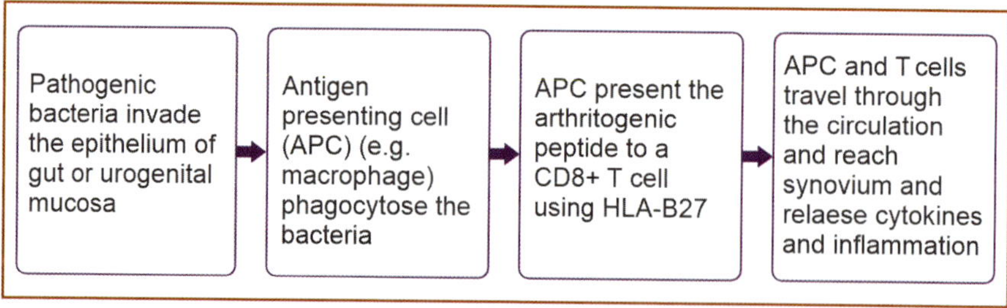

Fig. 11.1: Mechanism of reactive arthritis

Table 11.1: Bacteria associated with the development of reactive arthritis

Common causative agents

Enteric infections	Urogenital infections
Salmonella	*Chlamydia trachomatis*
Various serovars	*Ureaplasma urealyticum*
Shigella	*Mycoplasma genitaliuma*
S. flexneri	Respiratory infections
S. dysenteriae	*Chlamydia pneumoniae*
S. sonnei	Group A beta-hemolytic Streptococcus
Yersinia	
Y. enterocolitica (especially O:3 and O:9)	
Y. pseudotuberculosis	
Campylobacter	
C. jejuni	
C. coli	
Clostridium difficile	
Escherichia coli	
Diarrhogenic strains	

Uncommon causative agents

B-haemolytic Streptococci	Intravesical Bacillus Calmette-Guerin (BCG)
Mycoplasma genitalium	*Neisseria gonorrhoea*
Ureaplasma urealyticum	*Staphylococcus aureus*
Chlamydia pneumoniae	*Staphylococcus epidermis*
Chlamydia psittaci	*Mycobacterium tuberculosis* (Poncet's disease)
Mycoplasma pneumoniae	COVID 19
HIV	

Clinical Features

Articular and Periarticular Symptoms

Acute asymmetrical oligoarthritis typically involves the large joints of the lower limb, especially the knee and talocrural joint. About 30% of patients experience enthesitis, commonly as plantar fasciitis or Achilles tendonitis. Sacroiliitis manifests as inflammatory back pain, and dactylitis is seen in around 40% of cases.

Mucocutaneous

Keratoderma blennorhagicum, which is characteristic of reactive arthritis (ReA), appears in about 20% of cases as pustular lesions on the plantar areas that can become scaly and hyperkeratotic. Circinate balanitis presents as painless, shallow psoriasiform lesions on the glans or shaft of the penis. Other manifestations include aphthous ulcers, onycholysis, and nail dystrophy.

Genitourinary Symptoms

Includes urethritis, cervicitis, salpingitis, pelvic inflammatory disease, epididymitis, orchitis, and prostatitis. Approximately 90% of patients experience either urethritis or cervicitis following a genitourinary infection.

Ophthalmological Manifestations

Conjunctivitis (most common), uveitis (second most common), episcleritis, scleritis, keratitis, optic neuritis, glaucoma, and retinal vasculitis.

Diagnosis

Diagnosis is essentially clinical. There are no validated diagnostic criteria but classification criteria were introduced in the 4th International Workshop on Reactive Arthritis (Table 11.2).

Other causes of acute arthritis (septic arthritis, crystal induced arthritis, acute rheumatic fever, viral infection) should be excluded.

Laboratory Testing

In cases of *Chlamydia trachomatis*, the infective organism can be isolated from urinary samples or urogenital swabs, however isolation from stool samples is not feasible, as arthritis typically develops after the resolution of enteric infections.

In acute ReA, both ESR and CRP levels are elevated. Ultrasound examination of the joints may reveal synovitis and tenosynovitis, while MRI is valuable for assessing sacroiliitis (Table 11.3).

Table 11.2: Braun criteria for reactive arthritis	
Major criteria	1. Arthritis with 2 or 3 of the following: • Asymmetric • Mono- or oligoarthritis • Predominantly affecting the lower limbs 2. Preceding symptomatic infection with 1 or 2 of the following: • Enteritis (diarrhea for at least 1 day, 3 days to 6 weeks before onset of arthritis). • Urethritis (dysuria or discharge for at least 1 day, 3 days to 6 weeks before the onset of arthritis).
Minor criteria, at least one of the following	1. Evidence of triggering infection: • Positive nucleic acid amplification test in the morning urine or urethral/cervical swab for *Chlamydia trachomatis*. • Positive stool culture for enteric pathogens associated with ReA. 2. Evidence of persistent synovial infection (positive immunohistology or PCR for Chlamydia).
Definition of reactive arthritis	• **Definite ReA:** both major criteria and a relevant minor criterion • **Probably ReA:** (a) both major criteria, but no relevant minor criteria or (b) major criterion 1 and one or more of the minor criteria

Table 11.3: Biologic agents studied in ReA		
	Drug	*Efficacy and safety*
Anti TNF agents	Infliximab	Yes
	Etarnacept	Yes
	Adalimumab	Yes
Interleukin 6 receptor antibody	Tocilizumab	Yes
Interleukin 17 A monoclonal antibody	Secukinumab	Yes

Treatment

Initial goals of therapy is to provide symptomatic relief and prevent chronic complications (Fig. 11.2).

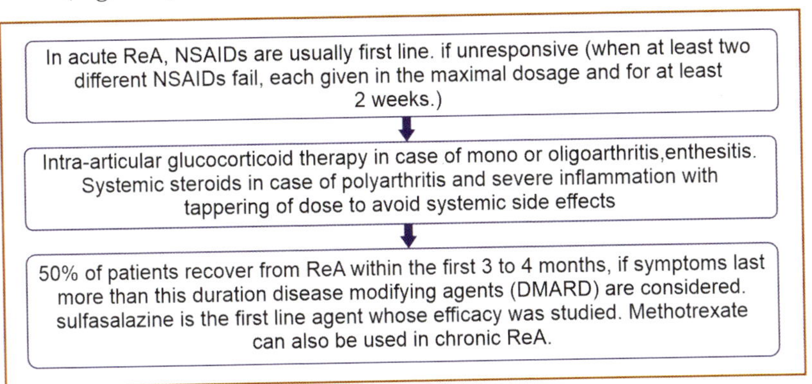

Fig. 11.2: Treatment of reactive arthritis

Prognosis

Average duration of acute ReA is 3–5 months. Arthritis lasting for >6 months is chronic and the factors determining chronicity are: Type of infection, presence of HLA-B27, positive family history for AS or SpA, and presence of chronic gut inflammation .

Clinical snippet

A 37-year-old woman presented with history of pain and swelling in right knee, left ankle swelling of left 5th toe, for 3 weeks associated with fever. One month before the onset of arthritis, she experienced diarrhea and denied any history of rash, ocular symptoms, or genitourinary issues. On examination, her left ankle and right knee were warm, tender, and swollen, with limited range of motion. Her CRP was 58 mg/L (normal 0–5 mg/L), WBC 11.5 (normal 4.5 to 11.0 × 109/L), HLA-B27 was negative, she was started on NSAID along with sulfasalazine. On follow up she was off NSAID and DMARD was continued with significant improvement in articular symptoms.

FURTHER READING

1. Henning Zeidler & Alan P. Hudson, Reactive Arthritis Update: Spotlight on New and Rare Infectious Agents Implicated as Pathogens, Current Rheumatology Reports (2021)23:53.
2. Ibtissam Bentaleb & Kawther Ben Abdelghani & Samira Rostom, Reactive Arthritis: Update, Current Clinical Microbiology Reports 2020.

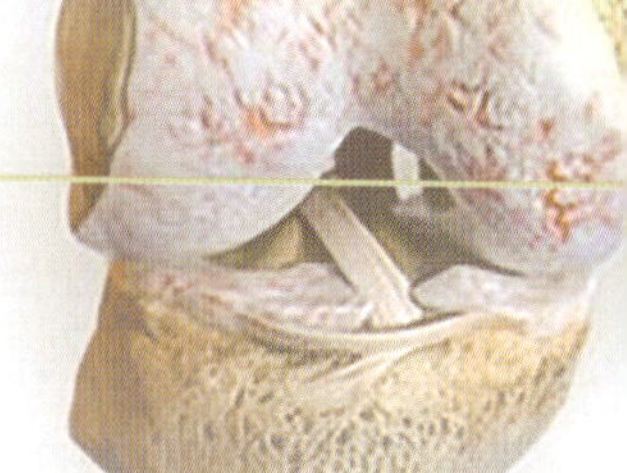

Inflammatory Bowel Disease-Associated Arthritis

P Sree Sanjay, Damodaram

INTRODUCTION

Arthritis associated with bowel diseases are called enteropathic arthritis. They are predominantly associated with IBD, both ulcerative colitis and Crohn's disease. However, enteropathic arthritis also includes other rare forms associated with Whipple disease, celiac disease and Intestinal bypass surgery associated arthritis. (1) Other inflammatory conditions that affect bowel and joints include Behçet's syndrome, familial Mediterranean fever (FMF) and yao syndrome. The classic Yao syndrome presents with recurrent fever, dermatitis, arthritis, distal extremity swelling, GI symptoms, and sicca-like symptoms/eyelid swelling. Most of the GI symptoms are of intermittent abdominal pain, bloating, and diarrhea. The current chapter will focus on IBD associated arthritis which is classified under the spectrum of spondyloarthritis.

Clinical Features

IBD associated arthritis can present as both peripheral arthritis and axial arthritis. The peripheral arthritis affects large joints such as knees, ankles, elbows, and wrists. The presentation is monoarticular, predominantly affecting knees or ankles. The disease can be oligoarticular, which is most often asymmetrical predominantly involving lower limb joints (also called Type 1 IBD associated arthritis). Rarely, IBD associated arthritis can also present in a symmetrical fashion involving both upper and lower limb joints similar to rheumatoid arthritis (also called Type 2 IBD associated arthritis). In such cases the already established IBD clinches the diagnosis and these patients are seronegative for rheumatoid factor (RF) and antibodies to citrullinated peptides (ACPA). The seronegative arthritis without intestinal manifestations can pose a challenge to differentiate it with seronegative rheumatoid arthritis. Type 1 arthritis is most often seen in the Crohn's disease than ulcerative colitis (6.0% vs 3.6%) and most often associated with other extraintestinal manifestations such as erythema nodosum and scleritis. Type 1 arthritis can present before IBD presentation in 30% of patients and most often self-limiting. It most commonly involves lower limb joints and deformities are uncommon. Type 1 is most often associated with HLAB27 and B35. Type 2 peripheral arthritis is also most often seen in Crohn's disease (4.0% vs 2%) and this variety most often correlates with intestinal disease activity and tends to be recurrent and more persistent than type 1. This is most often associated with HLA B 44.

Joint erosions and deformities can be seen in this group and not much associated with other extraintestinal manifestations except uveitis.

Axial arthritis involves the spine and sacroiliac joints. These patients can present with symptoms of inflammatory back pain, stiffness, particularly in the morning and prompt relief with non-steroidal anti-inflammatory drugs or get relieved with resumption of daily activities. In patients with symptoms of spondyloarthritis the presence of chronic diarrhea, pain abdomen, nocturnal diarrhea, unexplained weight loss, rectal bleeding not explained by hemorrhoids, perianal fistula and recurrent aphthosis can be potential clues for the underlying IBD. Conversely the presence of IBP, dactylitis, peripheral arthritis and enthesitis are potential clues for the development of spondyloarthritis in patients with IBD.

Diagnosis

Diagnosis is primarily clinical, supported by imaging studies such as X-rays, MRI, and ultrasound. Blood tests may show elevated inflammatory markers like ESR and CRP. X-rays can show sacroiliitis of different grades. The X-ray of peripheral joints may not show significant juxta-articular osteopenia and instead new bone formation can be noted at the periphery. MRI helps in the detection of peripheral arthritis and bone marrow edema and detect early spondyloarthritis manifestation before radiological visible damage. Ultrasound can detect subclinical enthesitis and peripheral arthritis. Colonoscopy and biopsy of intestinal lesions are crucial in confirming IBD in those patients who present predominantly with arthritis. It can also detect subclinical gut inflammation which is well prevalent in all forms of spondyloarthritis indicating early intestinal dysbiosis and gut inflammation. The elevated faecal calprotectin levels also suggest intestinal inflammation but is not very specific for IBD.

Treatment

The primary goal of the treatment is the control of the symptoms, high quality of life, minimising the long-term structural damage, preservation of the function and social life. The treatment consists of non-pharmacological and pharmacological therapies, The pharmacological therapies consist of nonsteroidal anti-inflammatory drugs (NSAIDs), disease-modifying antirheumatic drugs (DMARDs), such as methotrexate and sulfasalazine, are used for peripheral arthritis. The use of biological revolutionised the treatment of spondyloarthritis. In the presence of IBD, infliximab or adalimumab are more preferred than etanercept. Biologicals work both for axial and peripheral arthritis. Anti IL17 treatment is better avoided in IBD patients as it exacerbates the underlying IBD (Table 12.1). In contrast the small molecules such as tofacitinib are more effective in

Table 12.1: Summary of treatment options for IBD associated arthritis				
Medication	Crohns	Ulcerative colitits	Axial disease	Peripheral arthritis
NSAIDs	Avoid in active disease	Avoid in active disease	+	+
Systemic glucosteroids	+	+	-	-
Methotrexate	+			+
Sulfasalazine	+	+		+

(Contd.)

(Contd.)

Medication	Crohns	Ulcerative colitits	Axial disease	Peripheral arthritis
Infliximab	+	+	+	+
Etanercept			+	+
Ustakinumab	+	+	+	+
Secukunimab	avoid	Avoid	+	+
Tofacitinib		+	+	+

IBD arthritis as it controls both arthritis and IBD manifestations particularly ulcerative colitis, though dose is higher than that used in rheumatoid arthritis. In some cases, it may require a multidisciplinary approach, involving gastroenterologists, rheumatologists, and primary care providers.

FURTHER READING

1. Barkhodari, Amir, Lee, Kate E, Shen, Min, Shen, Bo and Yao, Qingping. "Inflammatory bowel disease: focus on enteropathic arthritis and therapy" *Rheumatology and Immunology Research*, vol. 3, no. 2,2022,pp.69–76.
2. Ramiro S, Nikiphorou E, Sepriano A, Ortolan A, Webers C, Baraliakos X, Landewé RBM, Van den Bosch FE, Boteva B, Bremander A, Carron P, Ciurea A, van Gaalen FA, Géher P, Gensler L, Hermann J, de Hooge M, Husakova M, Kiltz U, López-Medina C, Machado PM, Marzo-Ortega H, Molto A, Navarro-Compán V, Nissen MJ, Pimentel-Santos FM, Poddubnyy D, Proft F, Rudwaleit M, Telkman M, Zhao SS, Ziade N, van der Heijde D. ASAS-EULAR recommendations for the management of axial spondyloarthritis: 2022 update. Ann Rheum Dis. 2023 Jan;82(1):19–34.

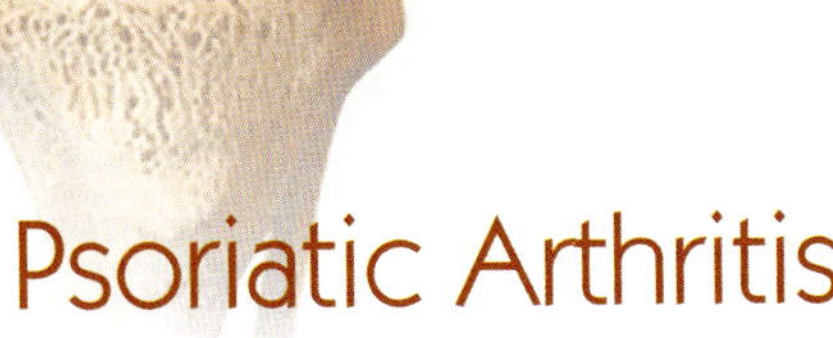

Psoriatic Arthritis

Bimlesh Dhar Pandey

INTRODUCTION

Psoriatic arthritis (PsA) is chronic inflammatory arthropathy associated with psoriasis (PsO). One-third of patients with psoriasis (PsO) develop psoriatic arthritis (PsA) at any given point in time. It is a complex disease characterised by multiple domains and features which often overlap between rheumatoid arthritis, osteoarthritis and spondyloarthritis (SpA).The credit of clinical expression of psoriasis and associated arthritis goes to alibertin his seminal paper way back in 1818[1]. PsA is now considered to be a part of SpA.

Clinical Features

When to suspect PsA in patient with PsO.
a. Nail involvement
b. Familial history of PsA
c. Obesity
d. History of arthralgias in patient with PsO
e. Psoriasis severity
f. Enthesial pain historically/ultrasound/MRI evidence of enthesitis

What constitutes PsA or Disease domains

a. **Peripheral Arthritis:** Usually involvesknees, elbows, wrists, MCP, PIP and DIP and feet. It can oligoarthritis which is 4 or less joints an early phenomenon versus polyarthritis which is 5 or more joint involvement as a late phenomenon. Radiographic joint damage can be seen in 50% of patients with PsA as early as 2 years from onset. Unique radiographic features also include new bone formation, bony ankylosis, and joint osteolysis.

b. **Enthesitis:** Inflammation of the entheses which is the interface where tendons, ligaments, and joint capsules gets attached to bone. Up to one-third of patient have enthesitis. The common areas include tendo-Achilles and plantar fascia insertions. Enthesitis may the first phenomenon before clinical synovitis. Chronic enthesitis causes bony spurformation and is called enthesophytes at peripheral sites and in axial spine it is known as syndesmophytes. Enthesitis contributes to pain and poor quality of life. Enthesitis can be assessed by MRI/musculoskeletal ultrasound.

c. **Dactylitis:** Diffuse swelling of an entire finger or toe, giving it a sausage-like appearance. 2nd and 3rd digit of the dominant hand or the 4th toe is the most common digits involved. It is the inflammation of tendons, entheses, soft tissue and synovitis involving MCP, PIP, and DIP joints. 50% of PsA may have dactylitis. It is considered to be marker of disease activity and progression with variable course.

d. **Nail psoriasis:** Includes pitting, crumbling, loosening ofthe nail plate discoloration, splinterhaemorrhage of the nail bed. It is a fore runner of PsA. It is also marker of disease activity.

e. **Axial disease:** Inflammatory back pain the hall mark feature. Has certain unique feature including equal gender association, asymmetrical syndesmophyte formation, early cervical spine involvement.

f. **Inflammatory bowel disease (IBD):** It is seen up to 4% of patients with PsA and is closely associated with severity of PsA.

g. **Uveitis:** Can be seen in a small sub set of patient of PsA and is again a marker of severity of PsA. It can cause variable vision morbidity.

Diagnosis

The original classification criteria by Moll and Wright[2] included
a. Asymmetrical oligoarthritis
b. Symmetrical polyarthritis
c. Distal interphalangeal joint (DIP) predominant arthritis
d. Arthritis mutilans
e. Spondylitis

Classification criteria should not be used as a diagnostic criteria. There are no diagnostic criteria for PsA.The scoring tool of classification criteria for psoriatic arthritis (CASPAR) has been a great help in uniformity of classifying patients with PsA.

Evidence of PsO	Points
Current PsO	2
History of PsO	1
Family history of PsO	1
Nail PsO	1
Negative rheumatoid factor	1
Dactylitis (current or past)	1
Radiologic evidence of juxta-articular bone formation	1

Score of ≥ 3 is considered to be significant and meets the criteria of PsA.
How to screen PsA in a busy OPD using validated PEST questionnaire.

Have you ever had a swollen joint/joints?	Yes	No
Has a doctor ever told you that you have arthritis?	Yes	No
Do your finger nails and toe nails have holes or pits?	Yes	No
Have you had pain in your heel	Yes	No
Have you had a finger or toe that was completely swollen and painful for no apparent reason	Yes	No

A score of 3 and above is considered positive and indicative of a requirement of consultation with a rheumatology expert.

Treatment

Objective: Individualised treatment protocol with objectivity of low disease state or remission, ensuring good quality of life and prevent complications associated with disease.

The concept of minimal disease activity (MDA) ensures the patient to have
a. Swollen joint count <1/66
b. Tender joint count <1/68
c. Psoriasis area and severity index (PASI)<1
d. Patient pain VAS <15
e. Patient global activity VAS <20
f. HAQ <0.5
g. Tender enthesial point <1

Background Health Assessment Prior to Initiation of Treatment

Disease Considerations	Practical Advice
Cardiovascular diseases	Optimum blood pressure management Tight lipid control Smoking cessation
Liver diseases	Assessment of fatty liver state and viral markers in an appropriate situation
Kidney diseases	Avoid NSAIDs
Diabetes	Tight control of blood sugar
Depression and anxiety	Avoid aprimilast Psychiatric assessment if required
Obesity	Ensure weight loss in obese patients

Assessment of disease domain and structured treatment (modified GRAPPA PsA Recommendations, 2021)

	Peripheral Arthritis	Axial Disease	Enthesitis	Dactylitis	Psoriasis	Nail Disease	IBD	Uveitis
First Line agent	csDMARDs methotrexate, leflunomide, sulphasalazine	NSAIDs	NSAIDs	NSAIDs, csDMARDs	csDMARDs, phototherapy	csD-MARDs	MTX	MTX
Second Line agent	TNFi, IL-17i, JAKi, PDE4i	TNFi, IL-17i, JAKi,	MTX TNFi, IL17i, JAKi, PDE4i	MTX TNFi, IL17i, JAKi, PDE4i	TNFi, IL-17i, JAKi, PDE4i	TNFi, IL-17i, JAKi, PDE4i	TNFi, JAKi	TNFi, JAKi
Third Line agent	Switch biological JAKi PDE4i	Switch biological JAKi	Switch biological JAKi PDE4i	Switch biological JAKi PDE4i	Switch biological JAKiPDE4i	Switch biological PDE4i	IL12/23i IL-12i	Switch TNFi

Practical Tips and Safety Consideration

Drug name	Dosage	Toxicity
Methotrexate	15–30 mg/week. Oral/subcutaneous/Intramuscular Not safe during pregnancy	Baseline LFT. CBC and KFT. Bone marrow suppression and transaminitis
Leflunomide	20 mg once a day Not safe during pregnancy	Bone marrow suppression, transaminitis, weight loss, BP elevation
Cyclosporine	3–6 mg/kg/day Safe during pregnancy	Bone marrow suppression, kidney dysfunction, hypertension, gum hypertrophy
Sulphasalazine	2–3 gms/day Safe during pregnancy	Transaminitis, bone marrow suppression
JAKI (Tofacitinib)	5–10 mg/day Not safe during pregnancy	Increase risk of viral infection including herpes zoster, bone marrow and liver dysfunction
Apremilast (PDE4 I)	Up to 60 mg/day Not safe for pregnancy	Diarrhea, increased depression, and suicidal indentations
TNFi (etanercept, adalimumab, golimumab, infliximab)	Safe for pregnancy up to 2nd trimester	Increased risk of infection including tuberculosis/viral infections, fungal and bacterial infections)
IL-17i (secukinumab)	Induction 150 mg (subcutaneous) weekly for 5 doses, then maintenance once a month (not recommended during pregnancy)	Diarrhea, increased fungal infections, pharyngitis

Outcome in psoriatic arthritis depends on multiple clinical domains, correct assessment of disease activity periodically with background comorbidities and timely intervention.

FURTHER READING

1. Alibert J. Precis theorique et pratique sur les maladies de la peau. Paris: Caille et Ravier; 1818.
2. Moll JM, Wright V. Semin Arthritis Rheum. 1973;3:55–78
3. Kimak A, Robak E, Makowska J, Woźniacka A. Psoriatic arthritis: development, detection and prevention: a scoping review. Journal of Clinical Medicine. 2023 Jun 5;12(11):3850.
4. Coates, L.C., Soriano, E.R., Corp, N. et al. Group for Research and Assessment of Psoriasis and Psoriatic Arthritis (GRAPPA): updated treatment recommendations for psoriatic arthritis 2021. Nat Rev Rheumatol 18, 465–479 (2022). https://doi.org/10.1038/s41584-022-00798-0.

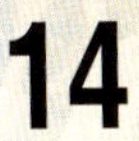

Sjögren's Syndrome

Sham Santhanam

INTRODUCTION

Sjögren's syndrome (SS) is a chronic autoimmune disease named after Swedish ophthalmologist Henrik Sjögren, who reported a case series of keratoconjunctivitis sicca with salivary gland enlargement in a few of them. These patients present with mouth dryness (xerostomia) and ocular dryness (xerophthalmia) due to immune-mediated damage of the salivary and lacrimal glands. This can extend to the airways, the esophagus, and even the vagina leading to the 'sicca complex' or 'sicca syndrome'. Sjögren's syndrome is a systemic disease and can practically involve any of the other organ systems, leading to the less common extraglandular manifestations like arthritis, peripheral neuropathy, etc. It can be defined as 'primary' in isolation or 'secondary' when associated with other connective tissue disorders like systemic lupus erythematosus, rheumatoid arthritis or systemic sclerosis.

Clinical Features

The clinical features of Sjögren's syndrome can be divided into glandular and extra-glandular manifestations. Though more than 50% of patients can develop extraglandular features, only 15% develop severe features.

a. **Glandular features:** The common symptoms are ocular dryness (photosensitivity, grittiness of eyes), mouth dryness (difficulty in speaking for a long time, altered taste, dysphagia, pain and burning sensation), respiratory tract dryness (dry cough, hoarseness of voice), dry skin and vaginal dryness (dyspareunia). On examination, they can have features of salivary gland enlargement, dental caries, fissured tongue, oral candidiasis, de-papillated or fissured tongue and red eyes.

b. **Extraglandular features:** Musculoskeletal involvement: Arthritis (non-erosive, symmetric)

   Dermatological: Besides xerosis, they can have purpura, annular erythema, cutaneous vasculitis (as ulcers, urticarial vasculitis, nodules), and Raynaud's syndrome.

   Pulmonary: Interstitial lung disease [non-specific interstitial pneumonia (more common), lymphoid interstitial pneumonia (typical for SS, but rare)], organizing pneumonia, follicular bronchiolitis, bronchus-associated lymphoma, and pulmonary artery hypertension.

Neurological: Peripheral nervous system (symmetric peripheral neuropathy, painful small fiber neuropathy, autonomic neuropathy, cranial neuropathy) involvement is more common than central nervous system (minor cognitive, mood disturbances, focal CNS disturbances) involvement, which can be associated with neuromyelitis optica (NMO spectrum disorders).

Renal: Chronic tubulointerstitial nephritis, distal renal tubular acidosis

Gastrointestinal: Dysphagia, motility disorders, exocrine pancreatic dysfunction and abnormal liver function tests due to associated various disorders (autoimmune hepatitis, primary biliary cirrhosis) including coeliac disease.

Constitutional symptoms: Fatigue, fever (rare), sleep disorders, anxiety, depression and fibromyalgia-like symptoms (SS always need to be excluded before diagnosing someone with fibromyalgia)

Patients with SS are at increased risk for cardiovascular and cerebrovascular events. Non-Hodgkin's lymphoma is one of the severe complications associated with SS, and the risk factors are mentioned in Box 14.1.

Diagnosis

The diagnosis of SS needs a combination of subjective and objective findings with a high index of suspicion (Box 14.2). The 2016 American College of Rheumatology/European League Against Rheumatism Classification Criteria for Sjögren's syndrome is the recent criteria used to classify it as SS (Table 14.1). If minor salivary gland biopsy (MSG) is not possible, ultrasonography of the salivary gland can be a useful tool in the

Box 14.1: Risk factors for lymphoma
Salivary gland enlargement
Lymphadenopathy
Raynaud's phenomenon
Anti-Ro/La antibodies
Rheumatoid factor positivity; cryoglobulinemia
Monoclonal gammopathy
Low C4 (complement) levels [most predictive]

Box 14.2: When to suspect Sjogren's syndrome?
Sicca symptoms/severe dental caries
Fibromyalgia-like clinical presentation
Rheumatoid factor +ve with Anti CCP -ve
Hypergammaglobulinemia
Hypokalemic periodic paralysis
Medullary nephrocalcinosis
Small fibre neuropathy
Lymphoid interstitial pneumonia

Table 14.1: 2016 American College of Rheumatology/European League Against Rheumatism Classification Criteria for Sjögren's syndrome

Item	Score
Minor salivary gland lip biopsy—foci score ≥1	3
Serology—presence of Anti-Ro/SS-A antibodies	3
Ocular staining score [≥5 using lissamine green and fluorescein dye or ≥4 with Rose Bengal staining]	1
Schirmer's test ≤5 mm/5 minutes in at least one eye	1
Unstimulated whole salivary flow < 0.1 ml per minute	1

Rules for classification: Subjective symptoms of ocular or oral dryness with a total score of 4 or greater shall be classified as Sjögren's syndrome

Exclusion criteria: Head and neck radiation, active hepatitis C infection, acquired immunodeficiency syndrome; sarcoidosis, amyloidosis, graft versus host disease and IGG4 related disease

diagnosis of SS. Similarly, MSG biopsy is considered in practice when the clinical and serological features are not sufficient to make the diagnosis.

Treatment

The management of Sjögren's syndrome depends on the glandular and extraglandular manifestations and the severity of involvement. The drugs/strategies used in the treatment of SS are summarized in Table 14.2.

Clinical Snippet

A 52-year-old female presented with fatigue, polyarthralgia, dry mouth and purpuric lesions in both lower limbs. On examination, she had poor dental hygiene and enlarged parotid glands. On evaluation, she had leukopenia, elevated ESR, hypergammaglobulinemia, rheumatoid factor positivity and anti-CCP negativity.

Table 14.2: The various treatment options available for glandular and extraglandular manifestations of Sjögren's syndrome

Drug name	Dosage	Indications	Toxicity/Contraindications
Tear supplements	Low viscosity tears like drops in day time (4 times/day) High viscosity tears like gel at bed time	Dry eye	Preservative based tears may worsen dry eye; so increased frequency of applications warrants preservative free tear supplements
Topical cyclosporine[@]	0.05%-approved by FDA	Dry eye	Trouble tolerating the drops–have burning sensation
Pilocarpine[#]	5 mg three to four times daily	Dry mouth	Sweating, flushing, abdominal pain, diarrhea; contraindicated in iritis, narrow angle glaucoma and moderate to severe asthma
Topical fluoride salivary substitutes (hypromellose, methylcellulose)	4–6 times—moth gargling	Dry mouth	Limited benefit due to short duration of action
Clotrimazole cream, nystatin elixir, fluconazole/ clotrimazole troches	Topical application	Oral candidiasis due to severe dry mouth	In Sjögren's oral candidiasis may not be like typical white patch, it can be like atrophic glossitis.
Hydroxychloroquine	200–400 mg/day	Arthralgia, fatigue	Retinal toxicity; needs annual eye check up
Steroids immunosuppressives (MTX/AZA/MMF/ RTX)	Prednisolone (0.25–1 mg/kg/day) Dose of immunosuppressive agents depends on the type of drug	Organ threatening extraglandular manifestations like ILD, vasculitic neuropathy, interstitial nephritis	Depending on the agent–steroid or other immunosuppressives regular monitoring of blood counts, sugars, lipid profile, liver function tests need to be done at regular intervals to monitor for drug toxicity

@: Punctal occlusion (temporary followed by permanent occlusion) in patients with persistent dry eyes; #: Cevimeline is also helpful, but not available in India; MTX: Methotrexate; MMF: Mycophenolate mofetil; AZA: Azathioprine; RTX: Rituximab; similarly for dry skin and vaginal dryness moisturizers and topical creams are used.

She tested positive for ANA (1: 640; fine speckled, by indirect immunofluorescence) and had anti-SS-A, SS-B antibody positivity on the ANA profile (line immunoassay) method. She had severely dry eyes, and her Schirmer's was less than 5 mm in both eyes. Since a diagnosis of SS was made with clinical features, serological positivity, and objective evidence of dry eyes, there was not a need for an MSG biopsy. She was treated with tear supplements (dry eyes), pilocarpine, salivary substitute (dry mouth) and hydroxychloroquine (polyarthralgia) and improved symptomatically.

FURTHER READING

1. Mariette X, Criswell LA. Primary Sjögren's Syndrome. N Engl J Med. 2018 Mar 8;378(10):931–939. doi: 10.1056/NEJMcp1702514.

2. Shiboski CH, Shiboski SC, Seror R, Criswell LA, Labetoulle M, Lietman TM, et al. International Sjögren's Syndrome Criteria Working Group. 2016 American College of Rheumatology/European League Against Rheumatism Classification Criteria for Primary Sjögren's Syndrome: A Consensus and Data-Driven Methodology Involving Three International Patient Cohorts. Arthritis Rheumatol. 2017 Jan;69(1):35-45. doi: 10.1002/art.39859.

3. Seror R, Nocturne G, Mariette X. Current and future therapies for primary Sjögren syndrome. Nat Rev Rheumatol. 2021 Aug;17(8):475-486. doi: 10.1038/s41584-021-00634-x.

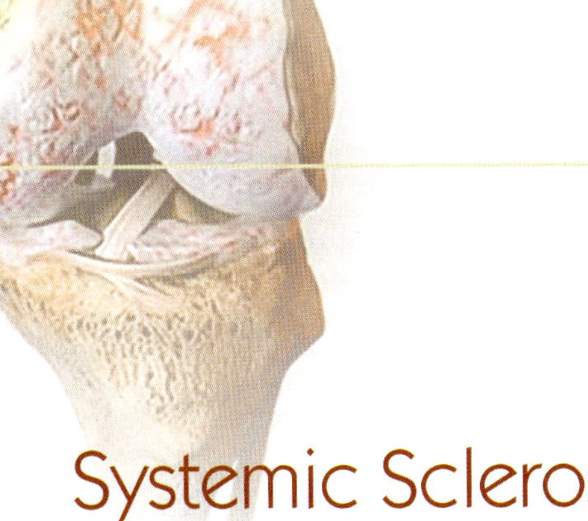

Systemic Sclerosis

Shabina Habibi

INTRODUCTION

Systemic sclerosis (SSc) is a chronic multisystem autoimmune disease, characterised by autoimmunity, vasculopathy, and fibrosis involving different organs.

Clinical Features

Patients are classified based on the extent of skin involvement and pattern of internal organ involvement into limited cutaneous(LcSSc) and diffuse cutaneous (DcSSc) subtypes. Patients without the characteristic skin thickening but having specific antibodies and internal organ manifestations are said to have systemic sclerosis *sine* scleroderma. SSc may overlap with other autoimmune disorders, classed as SSc overlap syndrome.

Cutaneous manifestations include skin thickening and hardening (proximal to the MCP joints), limited to face and below elbows/knees in the limited-subtype, and proximal to the above in diffuse-subtype. In early stages puffy/swollen fingers and non-pitting edema of the hands may be observed. Calcinosis cutis may be seen in advanced disease.

Digital vasculopathy resulting in Raynaud's phenomenon, with characteristic nail fold capillary dilation and dropout are observed years before other symptoms, particularly in the LcSSc subset. Other features include mucocutaneous telangiectasia, digital tip ulcers, scarring or gangrene due to digital ischemia.

Musculoskeletal manifestations include arthralgia, myalgia, arthritis, tendonitis, tendon friction rub(marker for severe disease with internal organ involvement) and joint contractures, especially involving fingers, due to fibrosis across tendons and the periarticular structures. Frank inflammatory arthritis with joint erosions is rare, except in overlap with rheumatoid arthritis.

Gastrointestinal manifestations occur due to involvement of the entire GI tract with fibrosis in 90% of patients and include dysphagia, reflux, heartburn, early satiety and bloating, diarrhea, constipation, pseudo-obstruction, bacterial overgrowth, faecal incontinence. Vascular ectasia in the gut wall can result in bleeding (usually chronic, rare acute) and anemia.

Pulmonary involvement is characterised by interstitial lung disease (ILD) (usually DcSSc), and pulmonary artery hypertension (PAH) (usually LcSSc). This causes breathlessness, reduced exercise tolerance, fatigue and right heart failure in advanced disease.

Cardiac involvement occurs due to ILD and PAH. All regions of the heart may however be affected.

Renal involvement by glomerulonephritis is rare. However, renal crisis resulting in malignant hypertension and renal failure can be seen in dcSSc.

Others include muscle wasting and weakness and sexual dysfunction in both men and women.

Diagnosis

Physical examination to look for puffy fingers, sclerodactyly, digital tip ulcers or scarring, peri-oral skin tightening with restricted mouth opening, calcinosis cutis, evidence of nutritional deficiencies due to GI involvement, etc. Cardiovascular examination for evidence of ILD (fine end inspiratory crepitations) or PAH(loud P2).

Laboratory testing: In addition to routine CBP, test for CK in patients with suspected overlap myositis, renal function and urine dipstick to detect early renal crisis. ANA is positive in >95% individuals with SSc. A negative ANA should therefore, prompt consideration of an alternative diagnosis. Certain ANA subsets point towards an increased risk of internal organ manifestations, e.g. anticentromere positive increases the risk of PAH, anti-topoisomerase antibodies of ILD, RNA polymerase III of renal crisis.

Testing for extracutaneous involvement is required to determine the extent of disease. Evaluation for ILD and PAH must be done for all patients. This includes pulmonary function test (PFT) to assess for restrictive ventilatory defect or decrease in single breath diffusion capacity for carbon monoxide (DLCO) and HRCT chest for ILD, and a baseline Echo for PAH.

Treatment

This should be started early in the disease course to reduce progression and subsequent damage. As the disease can involve different organs, management is tailored to the individual patient. Patients with severe or rapidly progressive disease are treated with aggressive immunosuppressive treatment. Since glucocorticoids are associated with an increased risk of renal crisis, they should be avoided or limited to short courses and low doses.

Clinical feature	Drug(s) used	Comments
Skin thickening	Methotrexate, mycophenolate mofetil	Limited/modest benefit
Refractory severe cutaneous sclerosis	IV Immunoglobulin, rituximab, tocilizumab, cyclophosphamide	
Raynaud's disease	Dihydropiridine calcium channel blockers such as nifedipine (30–120 mg/day). Alternatives include phosphodiesterase 5 inhibitors(sildenafil 20–40 mg 1–3 times a day), Losartan (50 mg/ day) or Fluoxetine (20 mg/day)	Conservative measures including woollen gloves and socks, maintaining warm core body temperatures, avoiding sudden changes in temperature, smoking cessation, avoid vasoconstrictors

(Contd.)

(Contd.)

Clinical feature	Drug(s) used	Comments
Digital ischemia and gangrene	IV Iloprost, epoprostenol Phosphodiesterase inhibitors-sildenafil, endothelin receptor antagonists-bosentan	
Associated inflammatory arthritis or myositis	Methotrexate, mycophenolate mofetil(MMF)	If cyclophosphamide used, MTX and MMF are not given
GI reflux	Proton pump inhibitors (Once or twice a day)	Others include H2 receptor antagonists, prokinetics
Bloating and early satiety		Non-pharmacological measures, including small frequent meals, avoiding fatty foods
Small intestinal bacterial overgrowth	Antibiotics	
Faecal incontinence	Bile acid binding resins, anti-diarrheal	Usually due to bacterial overgrowth and malabsorption
PAH	Calcium channel blockers, iloprost, bosentan, sildenafil, tadalafil	Supporting measures including smoking cessation, inotropes, oxygen, diuretics where appropriate
ILD	Mycophenolate(1.5–3 gm/day in two divided doses), Cyclophosphamide (CYP), Azathioprine (less efficacious than the above	Tocilizumab may be used in intolerance or when others contraindicated. MMF has better tolerability and comparable efficacy as CYP

Prognosis

There is an increased risk of mortality in these patients. ILD, PAH are the predominant causes of high mortality. Overall survival has improved in recent times. Male gender, younger age at onset, extensive cutaneous involvement, cardiopulmonary and renal disease and antibodies including anti-Topoisomerase and Th/To are associated with higher mortality risk.

Clinical Snippet

A 55-year-old lady with 1year of RP presents to her GP. She reports mild reflux symptoms and bloating. Examination reveals skin tightening over face and forearms, telangiectasia over face, restricted mouth opening. Cardiovascular, respiratory examinations are normal. Nail-fold capillaroscopy reveals capillary dilation and dropout.

Complete blood count shows mild normocytic anaemia. ESR and CRP are normal. ANA is positive at a titre of 1/640, with centromere pattern. Chest radiograph is normal. Baseline Echo shows mean pulmonary artery systolic pressure of 22 mmHg at rest, and PFT reveals DLCO of 95%.

She has LcSSc with GI involvement and PAH.

She is treated with calcium channel blockers and omeprazole, advised conservative measures for RP and reflux symptoms, and referred on to rheumatology.

FURTHER READING

1. Evidence-based detection of pulmonary arterial hypertension in systemic sclerosis: the DETECT study. Coghlan JG, Denton CP, Grünig E, et al. Ann Rheum Dis. 2014;73(7):1340.
2. Mycophenolate mofetil versus oral cyclophosphamide in scleroderma-related interstitial lung disease (SLS II): a randomised controlled, double-blind, parallel group trial. Tashkin DP et al. Lancet Respir Med. 2016;4(9):708.

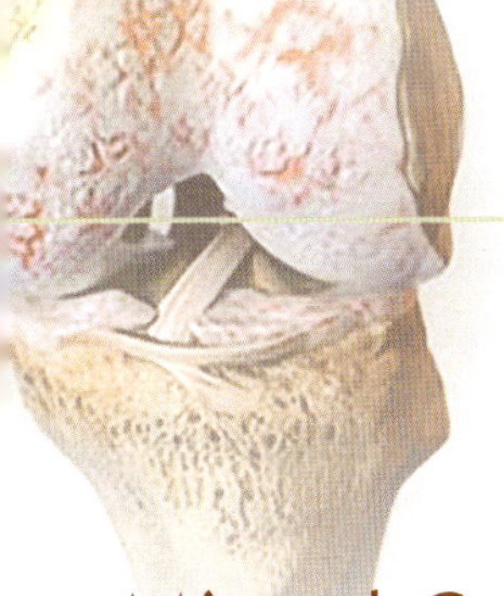

Mixed Connective Tissue Disease

Kavyasree Sunil, Nilesh Nolkha

INTRODUCTION

Mixed connective tissue disease (MCTD) is a distinct autoimmune disease with the main features of at least 2 overlapping connective tissue diseases, including systemic lupus erythematosus, systemic sclerosis, polymyositis, dermatomyositis, and rheumatoid arthritis. The reported prevalence of MCTD is 2–4 per 100,000 population. Unlike SLE, precipitation by sunlight and drug exposure has not been related to the onset of MCTD.

Clinical Features

Earlier in the course of disease, most patients complain of fatigue, poorly defined myalgias, arthralgias and Raynaud's phenomenon. A high titre of anti-RNP antibodies is a powerful predictor of evolution to MCTD.

Fever

Fever of unknown origin can be an initial presentation of MCTD and there can be co-existent myositis, aseptic meningitis, serositis or infections.

Bone and Joints

Joint pain and stiffness is an early symptom in nearly all patients. Classical Jaccoud's type of arthropathy has been described in MCTD, but erosive disease can occur with an associated ACPA positivity.

Skin and Mucous Membranes

Raynaud's phenomenon is the most common and one among the earliest manifestations. It may be accompanied by puffy and swollen digits.

Muscle

It varies from myalgia with no demonstrable weakness or EMG abnormalities with normal muscle enzymes to inflammatory myositis.

Blood Vessels

MCTD is often associated with capillary dilatation and drop out in nail-fold capillaroscopy. Bland intimal proliferation and medial hypertrophy is the characteristic vascular lesion in MCTD, which is the pathological basis for pulmonary hypertension and renovascular crisis.

Heart

Pericarditis is the most common cardiac manifestation reported in 10–30% of patients.

Lungs

Reported in 75% of cases. PAH is the most severe form of lung involvement. ILD occurs in as many as 50% of cases.

Renal

High titers of anti-U1RNP antibodies are relatively protective against the development of diffuse proliferative glomerulonephritis, regardless of whether they occur in a setting of classic SLE or MCTD. Renal changes are usually in the form of a membranous glomerulonephritis.

Gastrointestinal

Reported in approximately 60–80% of patients, most common being disordered motility in the upper GI tract. Abdominal pain in MCTD may result from bowel hypomotility, serositis or mesenteric vasculitis. Malabsorption syndrome can occur secondary to bacterial overgrowth.

Nervous System

CNS involvement is not classical in MCTD, most common being trigeminal neuralgia. Headaches are a relatively common symptom, vascular in origin in the majority of cases with many components of classic migraine.

Blood

Anemia is found in 75% of cases, usually anemia of chronic disease. Positive Coombs test has been documented in 60% of cases, but overt hemolytic anemia is uncommon. Lymphopenia has been documented in 75% of cases, correlates with disease activity.

Table 16.1: Diagnostic criteria for MCTD	
Alarcon-Segovia Criteria	*Kahn Criteria*
a. **Serological criteria** Anti-RNP at a hemagglutination titre of ≥1/1600.	a. **Serological criteria:** A high titre of anti-RNP corresponding to a speckled ANA of ≥ 1/1200 titre.

b. **Clinical criteria**
  1. Swollen hands
  2. Synovitis
  3. Myositis (biologically proven)
  4. Raynaud's phenomenon
  5. Acrosclerosis
	b. **Clinical criteria**
	  1. Swollen fingers
	  2. Synovitis
	  3. Myositis
	  4. Raynaud's phenomenon

MCTD present if criterion A is accompanied by three or more clinical criteria—one of which must include synovitis or myositis	**MCTD** present if criterion A is accompanied by Raynaud's phenomenon and two or more of the three remaining clinical criteria.

Treatment

Management of systemic manifestation and Raynaud's phenomenon is given in Tables 16.2 and 16.3.

Table 16.2: Management of systemic manifestations			
Drug Name	*Dose*	*Toxicity/ Contraindications*	*Special notes*
NSAIDs	Depending on the medication	Gastric Intolerance and ulcers. Cardiovascular risk. Contraindicated in CKD	Effective for arthritis and serositis.
Antimalarials Hydroxychloroquine	5 mg/kg/day	Skin pigmentation and rashes. Retinal toxicity	Effective for arthritic and cutaneous manifestations. Metabolic benefits
Methotrexate	7.5–25 mg/ week	Mucositis Myelosuppression	Effective for arthritis and skin manifestations, myositis and vasculitis.
Glucocorticoids	Varying-Low dose (up to 7.5 mg of prednisolone equivalent per day) to pulse methylprednisolone therapy (15–30 mg/kg for 3 consecutive days)	Gastric ulcers, Hypertension, Hyperglycemia, Cushingoid features, suppression of HPA axis, Osteoporosis, proximal myopathy	Autoimmune hemolytic anemia, thrombocytopenia, myositis, arthritis, vasculitis, myocarditis, pericarditis, interstitial lung disease, glomerulonephritis and nephrotic syndrome
Cyclophosphamide	Low dose Eurolupus regiemen — 500 mg IV every 2 weeks for 6 cycles. High dose NIH regimen — 500–750 mg/m^2 monthly for 6 cycles followed by 8 quarterly infusions.		
Azathioprine	2–3 mg/kg per day	Leukopenia, fever, rash, GI intolerance	Effective for mucocutaneous manifestations, ILD, renal, myositis and vasculitic manifestations
Mycophenolate Mofetil	2–3 g/day	Gastric intolerance, bone marrow toxicity, alopecia	Effective for mucocutaneous, ILD, renal, myositis and vasculitis

Table 16.3: Management of Raynaud's phenomenon			
Drugs	*Dosage*		*Common side effects*
CCB	Nifedipine	10–30 mg TID	Hypotension, Headache, edema, flushing and palpitation
	Nifedipine XL	30–60 mg TID	
	Amlodipine	5–10 mg OD	
	Felodipine	2.5–10 mg BID	

(Contd.)

(Contd.)

Drugs		Dosage	Common side effects
PDE-5 inhibitors	Sildenafil	20–15 mg TID or 50 mg BID	Hypotension, headache, flushing
	Tadalafil	20 mg OD to BID	
	Vardenafil	10 mg BD	
Prostanoids	Iloprost	0.5–2 ng/kg/min IV for 6–24 hr during 2–5 days monthly	Hypotension, headache, flushing, palpitation, arrhythmia, pulmonary edema
	Alprostadil	20 µg/hr IV for 3 hr during 5 days monthly	
	Epoprostenol	2 ng/kg/min IV infusion for 2–5 days	
ERA	Bosentan	62.5 to 125 mg BID PO	Hypotension, flushing, edema, headache

Prognosis

The prognosis for overlap syndromes is often better than for the classic AICTDs. Development of PAH or ILD is often associated with poor prognosis. Early diagnosis and prompt treatment may retard the progression of disease.

FURTHER READING

1. LeRoy EC, Maricq H, Kahaleh M. Undifferentiated connective tissue syndrome. *Arthritis Rheum* 23:341–343,1980.
2. Gaubitz M: Epidemiology of connective tissue disorders. *Rheumatology (Oxford)* 45(Suppl 3):iii3–iii4, 2006.
3. Vaz CC, Couto M, Medeiros D, et al: Undifferentiated connectivetissue disease: a seven-center cross-sectional study of 184 patients. *Clin Rheumatol* 28(8):915–921,2009.

Undifferentiated Connective Tissue Disease and Overlap Syndromes

Challa Madhuri

The complexity of autoimmune diseases is further compounded when a patient presents with symptoms related to more than one condition or when they occur in isolation. It thus becomes paramount to have a basic understanding of UCTD and overlap syndromes for non-rheumatology physicians.

UNDIFFERENTIATED CONNECTIVE TISSUE DISEASE

Introduction

Undifferentiated connective tissue disease (UCTD) is characterized by the presence of clinical symptoms and signs of autoimmune disease in addition to laboratory evidence of autoimmunity with the patients not fulfilling any of the widely used classification criteria for classic autoimmune diseases.

Clinical Features

The frequent clinical manifestations at onset are arthralgias (66%), arthritis (32%), Raynaud's phenomenon (38%), leukopenia (24%), xerostomia and xerophthalmia (21%), thrombocytopenia (9%), serositis (4%) and photosensitive rash (3%). Significant renal and neurological involvement is quite rare in UCTD.

Diagnosis

Though validated classification criteria for UCTD are not yet available, preliminary classification criteria have been proposed to distinguish between early and stable UCTD. Based on these criteria, UCTD is characterized by:

i. Signs and symptoms suggestive of a connective tissue disease, but not fulfilling the criteria for any defined CTDs

ii. Positive antinuclear antibodies, and

iii. A disease duration of at least 3 years. Patients with a shorter follow-up would be defined as having early UCTD. About 90–95% of the UCTD patients have positive ANA. Anti-Ro, anti-RNP, anti-dsDNA, and anti-phospholipid antibodies are seen in these patients in the same order of frequency.

Treatment

The most widely used drugs include NSAIDs, low-dose steroids, and antimalarial drugs like hydroxychloroquine. Methotrexate, azathioprine, and mycophenolate can be used as steroid-sparing agents according to the domain involved.

Prognosis

UCTD is a mild autoimmune condition with generally good outcomes. Around 25–30% of UCTD patients may evolve into a definite CTD especially during the first 2–5 years of symptom onset, while most remain undifferentiated. It is thus imperative to closely monitor these patients for any signs of evolution to a definite CTD, especially during major infections or pregnancy.

OVERLAP SYNDROMES

Introduction

Overlap syndrome is defined as meeting the criteria for more than one systemic autoimmune disease. The patients may develop features either simultaneously or sequentially. The classical example is mixed connective tissue disorder (MCTD), which is characterized by an overlap of clinical features of SLE, SSc, myositis, and RA. Whether MCTD should be thought of as a distinct entity or a subcategory of another condition like SLE or SSc remains a matter of debate. Other overlap syndromes include those with dominant features of systemic sclerosis or myositis, overlap of SLE and erosive deforming RA (termed rhupus) or with Sjögren's syndrome, overlap with autoimmune hepatobiliary diseases (like PBC) and autoimmune thyroid disorders.

Clinical Features

The most common clinical features in MCTD include hand edema, RP, arthritis, myositis, and sclerodactyly. NSIP pattern of ILD is seen in 50% of cases. PAH is an important cardiopulmonary manifestation. Profound neurological involvement is rare, but patients may experience headaches, trigeminal neuralgia, or polyneuropathy. Renal involvement is also relatively rare. Glomerulonephritis is typically membranous rather than proliferative. A scleroderma-like renal crisis has also been reported. Sicca, esophageal dysmotility, cytopenias, and serositis are other manifestations of MCTD/overlap syndromes. Patients with SSc-myositis overlap may have a higher prevalence of ILD and myocardial involvement.

Diagnosis

The typical patient with MCTD will have high titers of ANA with a speckled pattern. High titers of anti-U1RNP is required for the diagnosis of MCTD. Rheumatoid factor may be present in 50–75% and anti-Ro60 in around 30% of the patients. Though there are no internationally validated uniform diagnosed criteria for MCTD, the Alarcon-Segovia criteria is the most commonly used for research purposes amongst the several published criteria.

Anti-RNP Antibody Levels

Patients must have significantly elevated anti-Sm/RNP antibody levels, specifically an anti-U1 RNP titer greater than 1:1600.

Clinical Findings

Patients must also have at least three of the following clinical findings:
- Edema of the hands
- Synovitis
- Myositis
- Raynaud phenomenon
- Acrosclerosis/sclerodactyly

Other autoantibody associations in overlap syndromes have been summarized in Table 17.1.

Table 17.1: Autoantibody associations in overlap syndromes	
Auto-antibodies	*Clinical Features*
Anti U1-snRNP (MCTD)	SLE+ myositis +systemic sclerosis +RA
Anti PM-Scl	IIM+SSc-mechanics hands, sclerodactyly, RP and ILD
Anti-Ku and Anti-U3RNP	IIM+SSc
Anti-SSA/B + RF+ Anti-CCP	RA + Sjögren's

Treatment

Manifestation	*Drugs*	*Special notes*
Arthritis	NSAIDs, low dose steroids, methotrexate,	As in SLE, TNFi can potentially exacerbate disease in MCTD
Myositis	Steroids methotrexate/azathioprine/mycophenolate/rituximab	
RP Critical digital ischemia	CCBs, PDE5i, ERAs Heparin infusion, prostacyclin analogs. In refractory cases → Digital sympathectomy/Botox therapy	Cold protection measures must be followed
ILD	Mycophenolate, cyclophosphamide, rituximab	Annual PFT with DLCO monitoring
PAH	PDE5i or/and ERAs, selexipag, riociguat	Immunosuppression may have some benefit for MCTD related PAH.

Prognosis

The course of MCTD is varied, and many patients do follow a benign course. Severe renal involvement is uncommon. However, some patients have increased morbidity and mortality, with the most serious complication being PAH. SSc-myositis overlap patients may have increased mortality compared to SSc alone.

Clinical Snippet

A 40-year-old female had oral/ocular sicca, arthritis, and purpuric rashes. ANA was 4+S and Ro60 was strongly positive. Schirmer's test was 4 mm/3 mm in 5 minutes in the right/left eyes respectively. She was treated with LDS, HCQS and pilocarpine. 2 years later, she developed proteinuria with hypertension and low C3 and C4, renal biopsy showed class IV lupus nephritis. Thus, she was diagnosed with Sjögren's syndrome with SLE overlap and started on cyclophosphamide.

FURTHER READING

1. Pepmueller PH. Undifferentiated Connective Tissue Disease, Mixed Connective Tissue Disease, and Overlap Syndromes in Rheumatology. Mo Med. 2016 Mar-Apr;113(2):136–40.

2. Mosca M, Tani C, Bombardieri S. Undifferentiated connective tissue diseases (UCTD): a new frontier for rheumatology. Best Pract Res Clin Rheumatol. 2007 Dec;21(6):1011–23.

3. Nancy. J Olsen. Incomplete lupus, undifferentiated connective tissue disease, and mixed connective tissue disease In: DJ Wallace, BH Hahn eds. Dubois' Lupus Erythematosus and related syndromes. 10th ed. Philadelphia,PA: Elesevier;50,703–709.

4. Jonathan Graf.Overlap Syndromes Firestein & Kelley's Textbook of Rheumatology, 91,1569–1583. e4.

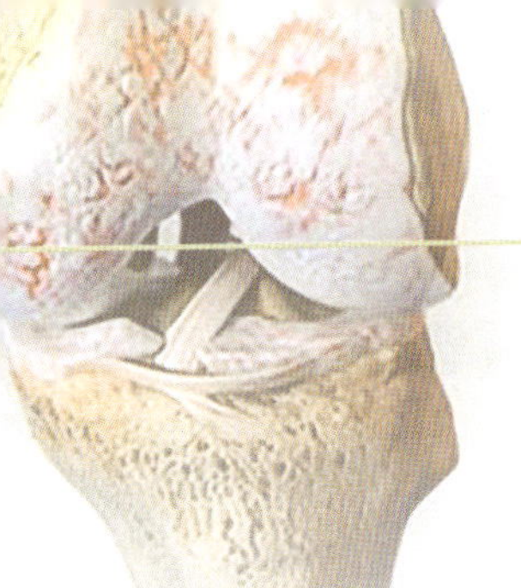

Inflammatory Muscle Disease

Ramya Janardana

Idiopathic inflammatory myositis (IIM) encompasses a heterogenous group of disorders which present with predominant proximal muscle weakness of varying degrees with or without skin rashes.

Historically two subsets of IIM, dermatomyositis (DM) and polymyositis (PM) were recognized, as early as 1975, when Bohan and Peter criteria for IIM diagnosis was published. Over the recent decades, with improving understanding of muscle pathology, multiple new myositis specific antibodies (MSAs) being discovered, new subsets such as inclusion body myositis, antisynthetase syndrome (ASS), immune mediated necrotizing myositis (IMNM), amyopathic dermatomyositis (ADM), overlap myositis have been described.

Epidemiology

Prevalence of IIM is around 14 in 1 lakh population, with dual peak (2–15 years and 45–60 years), almost equal gender ratio with the exception of overlap myositis (OM). IIM patients have 2 to 7 times increased risk of cancer, highest with dermatomyositis and lowest with overlap myositis.

Clinical features

IIM presents with subacute onset of proximal weakness, progressing over a few days or weeks to maximum weakness. The weakness is usually symmetrical involving proximal upper and lower limb muscles, truncal involvement is usual. Severe weakness is usually associated with bulbar weakness (dysphagia to solids, nasal regurgitation of feeds) and diaphragmatic weakness (shortness of breath, reduced breath holding time, reduced single breath count). Odd features are insidious onset of weakness, asymmetric involvement, involvement of ocular muscles, disproportionate atrophy and hypertrophy, disproportionate involvement of certain muscle groups (Table 18.1).

Presence of skin rash typical of DM is extremely useful for diagnosis. If there is a delay in presentation, look for faded rashes in the characteristic areas. Heliotrope rash, Gottron's sign and Gottron's papule are considered pathognomonic of DM. Heliotrope rash is typically described as violaceous erythema and edema over upper and lower eyelid. Depending on the ethnicity and skin pigmentation, the typical description may not be appreciated in all. Gottron's sign refers to macular erythema, Gottron's papules refer to raised erythematous lesion distributed over knuckles, elbows, sometimes over knee.

Table 18.1: Diagnosis and management of IIM					
Diagnosis	*Features in support of diagnosis*	*Pathological finding*	*Autoantibody*	*Treatment*	*Options in refractory disease*
Dermatomy-ositis	Subacute onset proximal muscle weakness with rash	Perifascicular atrophy is considered pathognomonic of DM. Other finding like perifascicular mononuclear cell infiltration, perifascicular necrosis, MxA deposition	MSAs such as Mi-2, TIF-1 gamma, SAE, NXP-2,MDA-5	High dose steroids with steroid sparing immunosuppression –methotrexate or azathioprine or mycophenolate or tacrolimus/ cyclosporine and Early initiation of exercises (resistance and strength training)	Intravenous immunoglo-bulins Rituximab
Polymyositis	Subacute onset proximal muscle weakness without rash	of CD 8+ T cell invasion of non-necrotic muscle fibers endomysial cells expressing MHC class I antigen	None	High dose steroids with steroid sparing immunosuppression –methotrexate or azathioprine or mycophenolate or tacrolimus/ cyclosporine and Early initiation of exercises (resistance and strength training)	Intravenous immunoglo-bulins Rituximab
Immune mediated necrotizing myositis	Acute to subacute in onset severe proximal muscle weakness, early atrophy		Anti SRP Anti HMG CoA reductase	Pulse steroids followed by high dose steroids and methotrexate IVIg in severe disease earlier use of rituximab if anti-SRP positive Early initiation of exercises (resistance and strength training)	Intravenous immunoglo-bulins Rituximab
Anti-synthetase syndrome and Overlap myositis	Subacute onset proximal muscle weakness without rash, raynaud's, skin tightness, sclerodactyly, mechanics hand	Perifascicular necrosis and some features of DM biopsies Perivascular mononuclear cells, scattered necrosis with sparse inflammation	Anti U1RNP Anti Ku Anti Pm-Scl Anti Jo-1 Anti Pl-7 Anti PL-12	High dose steroids with steroid sparing immunosuppression –methotrexate or azathioprine or mycophenolate or tacrolimus/ cyclosporine	Intravenous immunoglo-bulins Rituximab

(Contd.)

(Contd.)

Diagnosis	Features in support of diagnosis	Pathological finding	Autoantibody	Treatment	Options in refractory disease
Inclusion body myositis	Insidious onset, slowly progressive muscle weakness, early involvement of distal muscles especially finger flexors and atrophy of quadriceps and distal muscles, mild facial weakness, higher proportion of patients with dysphagia and axial involvement	Chronic myopathic changes, vacuoles and amyloid deposits detected by modified Gomori trichome and Congo red stain respectively	Anti C1Na	Recruitment into experimental therapy Early initiation of exercises (resistance and strength training)	Supportive care

The other rashes which are considered specific to DM are malar rash not sparing the nasolabial fold, V shaped erythema over upper chest (V sign), erythematous lesion over upper back (shawl sign), erythematous lesion over lateral thigh, cuticular irregularities, roughening of edges of palms and fingers (mechanics hand) and telangiectasias, generalized edema, poikiloderma, etc.

Involvement of extra-muscular organs, presence of features of CTD such as Raynaud's phenomenon, digital ulceration, sclerodactyly, skin tightness are also suggestive of a diagnosis of IIM (especially anti-synthetase syndrome/overlap myositis) in a patient presenting with proximal weakness. Interstitial lung disease (ILD) occurs in association with IIMPulmonary hypertension may be detected during evaluation of IIM.

Diagnosis

Classification criteria of IIM, typically incorporates historical aspects of muscle weakness, rashes, muscle enzyme elevation, biopsy features and electromyography findings.

The recent classification, ACR-EULAR IIM classification criteria has a weighted scoring for those with or without available muscle biopsy findings, classifies the diagnosis of IIM into definite, probable, possible based on the score, with greater sensitivity and specificity as compared to Bohan and Peter. Interestingly, although it incorporated a single MSA(Jo-1) into the criteria, it has omitted inclusion of many of the well established MSA (refer to Table 18.1).

Treatment

High dose corticosteroids are used during the initial course of active IIM. Dose may range from 0.5 mg/kg body weight to 1 mg/kg body weight with or without pulse methylprednisolone. Use of corticosteroid is based on clinical experience and small trials/retrospective data, however it remains the anchor drug in management of active IIM. Steroid taper as per clinician's experience and response.

Weekly low dose methotrexate as a steroid sparing agent has been used in the treatment of IIM for many decades now. The other steroid sparing immunosuppression used are azathioprine, mycophenolate mofetil, cyclosporine, tacrolimus depending on physician experience and extramuscular manifestations (mainly ILD).

Refractory IIM either cutaneous features or muscle disease can be managed with addition of intravenous immunoglobulins. There is recent trial data (ProDERM trial) as well to support this in DM patients. Rituximab can also be considered in refractory IIM patients, based on a large trial (RIM trial) conducted in refractory adult and juvenile IIM patients.

The above therapies are found to be ineffective for treatment of IBM over the long term. Symptomatic options are provided for worsening dysphagia and occasionally immunoglobulin therapy is offered.

FURTHER READING

1. Classification of IIM, pathological perspectives . Curr Opin Neurol 2019.
2. Alexander G S Oldroyd, et al, for the British Society for Rheumatology Standards, Audit and Guidelines Working Group, British Society for Rheumatology guideline on management of paediatric, adolescent and adult patients with idiopathic inflammatory myopathy, Rheumatology, Volume 61, Issue 5, May 2022.
3. Aggarwal R, et al, ProDERM Trial Group. Trial of Intravenous Immune Globulin in Dermatomyositis. N Engl J Med. 2022 Oct.
4. Oddis CV, et al, RIM Study Group. Rituximab in the treatment of refractory adult and juvenile dermatomyositis and adult polymyositis: a randomized, placebo-phase trial. Arthritis Rheum. 2013 Feb.

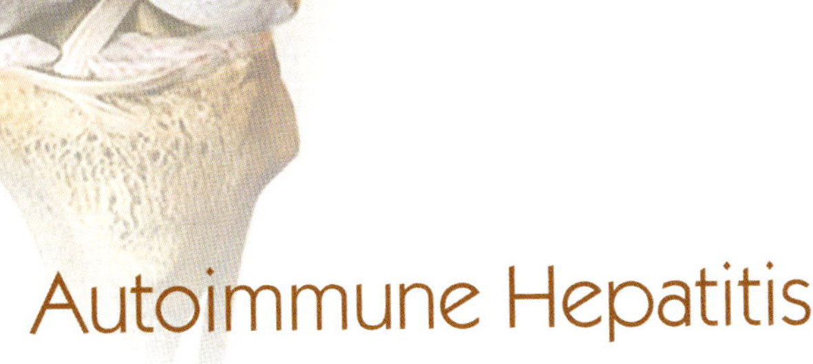

Autoimmune Hepatitis

Vikramraj K Jain

INTRODUCTION

Autoimmune hepatitis (AIH) is an immune mediated inflammatory liver disorder characterised by autoantibodies, raised IgG and specific biopsy findings. In a genetically predisposed individual and triggered by environmental factors the body's immune system mistakenly targets hepatocytes, leading to progressive liver inflammation and fibrosis. AIH can occur in individuals of all ages and races and in both sexes, although it is more common in women. Clinical features are heterogeneous ranging from asymptomatic disease to fulminant hepatic failure. Left untreated, AIH can progress to cirrhosis and liver failure, making early diagnosis and management critical.

Clinical Features

Autoimmune hepatitis usually presents with three patterns—acute, insidious and asymptomatic.

a. Acute onset is the most common pattern worldwide, presenting with transaminitis [5–10 times upper limit of normal], jaundice and raised international normalized ratio. Serum immunoglobulin G [IgG] levels are usually raised with typical autoantibodies and biopsy features of interface hepatitis. Some of them may progress to acute liver failure.

b. Insidious onset present with non-specific symptoms like arthralgia, fatigue, amenorrhea and sometimes with features of hepatic cirrhosis.

c. Asymptomatic form is usually found incidentally often in context of other autoimmune diseases.

A small proportion present with concomitant cholestatic features suggestive of overlapping primary biliary cirrhosis (PBC) or primary sclerosing cholangitis (PSC). Overlap PSC should be especially considered in patients with inflammatory bowel disease [especially ulcerative colitis] or those unresponsive to standard immunosuppressive treatment.

Diagnosis

The diagnosis of autoimmune hepatitis is based on a combination of clinical, laboratory, and histological findings. Any patient with unexplained elevated liver enzymes and/

or liver cirrhosis of unknown origin should be evaluated for autoimmune hepatitis. A point-based International Autoimmune Hepatitis Group simplified diagnostic criteria includes autoantibodies, hypergammaglobulinemia, histology and exclusion of viral hepatitis.

International Autoimmune Hepatitis Group, simplified criteria for the diagnosis of autoimmune hepatitis. [Hennes EM et al. Hepatology. 2008]

Clinical feature	Points
ANA or SMA	
• ≥1:40	+1
• ANA or SMA ≥1:80 or LKM1 ≥1:40 or SLA-positive	+2
Serum IgG	
• >Upper limit of normal	+1
• >1.1 times upper limit of normal	+2
Histologic findings	
• Compatible with AIH	+1
• Typical of AIH	+2
Hepatitis viral markers	
• Negative	+2
Aggregate score without treatment	
• Probable AIH	≥6
• Definite AIH	≥7

Liver Biopsy: Histological evaluation of the liver is mandatory for confirming the diagnosis. AIH is characterized by:
- Interface hepatitis (inflammation at the portal-parenchymal interface)
- Lymphoplasmacytic infiltrates
- Lobular hepatitis and bridging fibrosis in advanced stages
- Emperipolesis
- Hepatocellular rosette formation

A biopsy also helps to assess the degree of liver damage and guides therapeutic decisions.

Exclusion of Other Causes: It is essential to rule out viral hepatitis, drug-induced liver injury, herbal medicines, Wilson disease, hemochromatosis, non-alcoholic steatohepatitis and other causes of chronic liver disease.

Treatment

The primary goal of treatment in autoimmune hepatitis is to achieve sustained remission and prevent disease progression. The standard approach includes:
1. **Immunosuppressive Therapy:**
   - *Corticosteroids:* Prednisone is the first-line therapy for AIH with response to steroids being universal. The initial dose is typically high (e.g., 40–60 mg/day), followed by gradual tapering.
   - *Azathioprine:* Often added as a steroid-sparing and maintenance agent, azathioprine reduces the need for long-term corticosteroid therapy, minimizing side effects.

Drug	Dose	Toxicity	Caution/Contraindication
Prednisone	Initial: 40–60 mg/day, Taper: 5–10 mg/week	Weight gain, diabetes, hypertension, osteoporosis, mood swings	Uncontrolled diabetes, osteoporosis, peptic ulcer disease
Azathioprine	1–2 mg/kg/day	Bone marrow suppression, nausea, vomiting, hepatotoxicity, risk of malignancy	Severe liver disease, thiopurine methyltransferase (TPMT) deficiency
Mycophenolate Mofetil	1–2 g/day	Diarrhea, leukopenia, infections, teratogenicity	Pregnancy, severe renal impairment
Tacrolimus	0.05–0.1 mg/kg/day	Nephrotoxicity, neurotoxicity, hypertension, diabetes	Uncontrolled hypertension, renal insufficiency
Cyclosporine	2.5–5 mg/kg/day	Nephrotoxicity, hypertension, hirsutism, gingival hyperplasia	Uncontrolled hypertension, renal insufficiency, malignancies

- *Alternative agents:* For patients intolerant to azathioprine or corticosteroids, other immunosuppressants, such as mycophenolate mofetil, tacrolimus, or cyclosporine, may be considered.
2. **Monitoring and maintenance:** Once remission is achieved, long-term maintenance therapy is required to prevent relapse. Corticosteroids are tapered to the lowest effective dose, and azathioprine or another agent is continued at a maintenance dose.
3. **Treatment of relapse:** Relapses are common in AIH and are typically treated by re-initiating or increasing corticosteroid therapy.
4. **Liver transplantation:** In cases of decompensated cirrhosis or acute liver failure unresponsive to medical therapy, liver transplantation may be needed. AIH patients have good post-transplant outcomes, although there is a risk of disease recurrence of 8–12% in first year and 36–68% after five years.

Prognosis

The prognosis of autoimmune hepatitis depends largely on the stage of the disease at diagnosis and the response to treatment. With appropriate treatment autoimmune hepatitis has an excellent prognosis with long term survival and a good quality of life.. Untreated autoimmune hepatitis can lead to liver failure and death within five years in most patients. Delayed diagnosis or inadequate treatment can lead to complications, such as liver failure, liver cirrhosis and hepatocellular carcinoma.

Clinical Snippet

A 40-year-old woman presents with fatigue, jaundice, and mild abdominal discomfort. Her liver function tests show elevated ALT and AST, with a slight increase in bilirubin. Serum IgG is elevated, and testing reveals positive ANA and ASMA. A liver biopsy confirms the presence of interface hepatitis with lymphoplasmacytic infiltration. She is diagnosed with autoimmune hepatitis and started on prednisone and azathioprine. Over the following months, her symptoms improve, and her liver enzymes normalize. She continues on a maintenance dose of azathioprine and is monitored for potential relapse.

FURTHER READING

1. Mack CL, Adams D, Assis DN, et al. Diagnosis and Management of Autoimmune Hepatitis in Adults and Children: 2019 Practice Guidance and Guidelines From the American Association for the Study of Liver Diseases. Hepatology 2020;72:671-722. doi:10.1002/hep.31065.
2. Muratori L, Lohse AW, Lenzi M. Diagnosis and management of autoimmune hepatitis. BMJ. 2023 Feb 6;380:e070201. doi: 10.1136/bmj-2022-070201. Erratum in: BMJ. 2023 Feb 10;380:p330. doi: 10.1136/bmj.p330. PMID: 36746473.

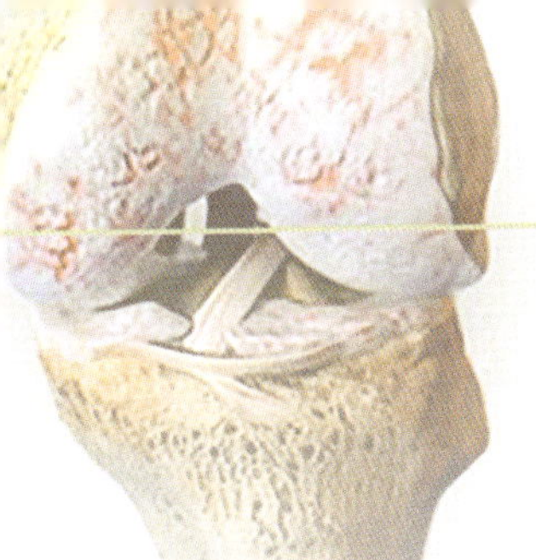

Shrinking Lung Syndrome

KV Kishore Babu

INTRODUCTION

Shrinking lung syndrome (SLS) is a rare pulmonary manifestation of systemic lupus erythematosus (SLE). It is very rarely reported in other systemic autoimmune diseases like systemic sclerosis, Sjögren's syndrome and rheumatoid arthritis. Prevalence of SLS is estimated to be between 0.5% and 1.1% in patients with SLE. Pathophysiology of SLS is largely unknown, many hypotheses have been proposed these include reduced diaphragmatic muscle thickness, diaphragmatic dysfunction due to pleural adhesions, pleural inflammation chronically impairing deep inspiration reducing lung compliance, paralysis of the phrenic nerve, alterations in surfactant, and myositis.

Clinical Features

SLS is typically suspected in patients with SLE who present with breathlessness on exertion, which progressed over several weeks to months, resulting in markedly decreased exercise tolerance and later dyspnea at rest, episodes of pleuritic chest pain, orthopnoea. Cough is less common, there may be reduced chest expansion, shallow and fast breathing. Lung auscultation usually normal or few basilar crepitations may be heard. Most of the patients do have extrapulmonary features of active SLE like arthritis, skin rashes, cytopenias, glomerulonephritis.

Diagnosis

There is no formal diagnostic criteria for SLS. It is a diagnosis of exclusion, and should be suspected in patients with typical presentation and combination of below features.

Unilateral or bilateral elevation of hemidiaphragm on radiograph. A few patients may have pleural effusions or pleural thickening.

Restrictive lung physiology on pulmonary function tests (PFT)- FVC <80% predicted and decreased DLCO.

No evidence of interstitial lung disease or significant pleural disease on radiograph or CT imaging.

Treatment

There are no evidence based guidelines for the management of SLS. Corticosteroids are the preferred first line agents. Usual dosage is 0.5 to 1 mg/kg of prednisolone per day, with subsequent tapering according to symptoms. A few patients may require pulse steroids depending on severity of SLS and extrapulmonary disease. Most of the patients demonstrate symptomatic improvement in chest pain and dyspnoea and increase in lung volumes in a few days to weeks. Inhaled beta-2 agonists, theophylline have been used as adjunctive therapy to improve diaphragmatic strength. Immunosuppressive agents such as cyclophosphamide, azathioprine, mycophenolate mofetil, and methotrexate have been tried in refractory cases with variable success. Rituximab was shown to be beneficial in steroid refractory patients in few case reports.

Prognosis

The prognosis for patients who have SLS is usually good, with most patients showing gradual improvement or stabilization of their pulmonary function.

FURTHER READING

1. Systemic lupus erythematosus in a multiethnic US Cohort LUMINA XLVIII: factors predictive of pulmonary damage. Bertoli AM, Vila LM, Apte M, et al. Lupus. 2007;16:410–417.
2. Singh R, Huang W, Menon Y, Espinoza LR. Shrinking lung syndrome in systemic lupus erythematosus and Sjögren's syndrome. J Clin Rheumatol. 2002 Dec;8(6):340–5.
3. Duron L, Cohen-Aubart F, Diot E, Borie R, Abad S, Richez C, Banse C, Vittecoq O, Saadoun D, Haroche J, Amoura Z. Shrinking lung syndrome associated with systemic lupus erythematosus: A multicenter collaborative study of 15 new cases and a review of the 155 cases in the literature focusing on treatment response and long-term outcomes. Autoimmun Rev. 2016 Oct;15(10):994–1000.

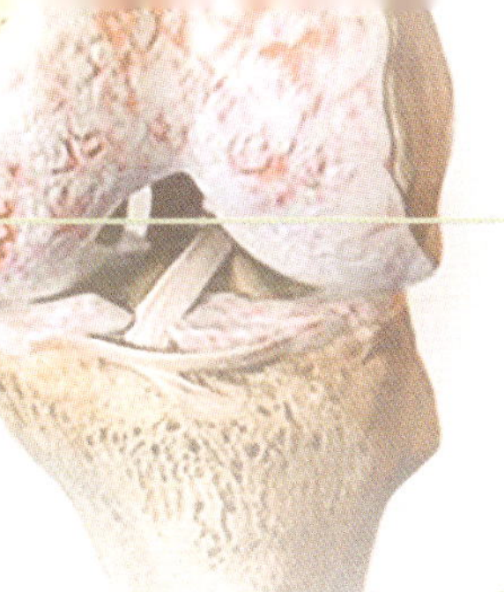

Interstitial Lung Disease

Srinivasa C

INTRODUCTION

Interstitial lung diseases (ILDs) encompass a diverse group of disorders characterized by inflammation and fibrosis of the lung parenchyma. These conditions arise due to various etiologies, including environmental exposures, autoimmune diseases, infections, and medications. Accurate diagnosis and management of ILDs require a multidisciplinary approach involving pulmonologists, radiologists, pathologists, and rheumatologists.

Diagnosis of ILDs

The diagnosis of ILDs begins with a comprehensive clinical history, physical examination, and laboratory tests. Common respiratory symptoms include progressive dyspnea, persistent cough, and exercise intolerance. Systemic features, such as arthralgia, rashes, fatigue, and Raynaud's phenomenon, may indicate an underlying autoimmune process.

Environmental and occupational exposures play a significant role in ILD etiology. Known risk factors include exposure to asbestos, silica, coal dust, cigarette smoke, bird antigens, and mold. Investigative measures include chest radiographs, pulmonary function tests, and high-resolution computed tomography (HRCT). In certain cases, bronchoalveolar lavage, transbronchial lung cryobiopsy, or surgical lung biopsy may be required to establish the diagnosis.

MAJOR SUBTYPES OF ILDs

Idiopathic Pulmonary Fibrosis (IPF)

IPF is a progressive fibrotic lung disease characterized by dyspnea, cough, and reduced exercise tolerance. HRCT typically reveals features of usual interstitial pneumonia (UIP), with reticular opacities, honeycombing, and lower-lobe predominance. The diagnosis is confirmed in the absence of alternative causes, such as connective tissue disease (CTD) or environmental exposures.

Histopathology of UIP shows temporal and spatial heterogeneity, architectural distortion, and fibroblastic foci. Guidelines recommend against invasive procedures for cases with a definite UIP pattern on HRCT, but bronchoalveolar lavage and biopsy may be necessary for probable or indeterminate patterns.

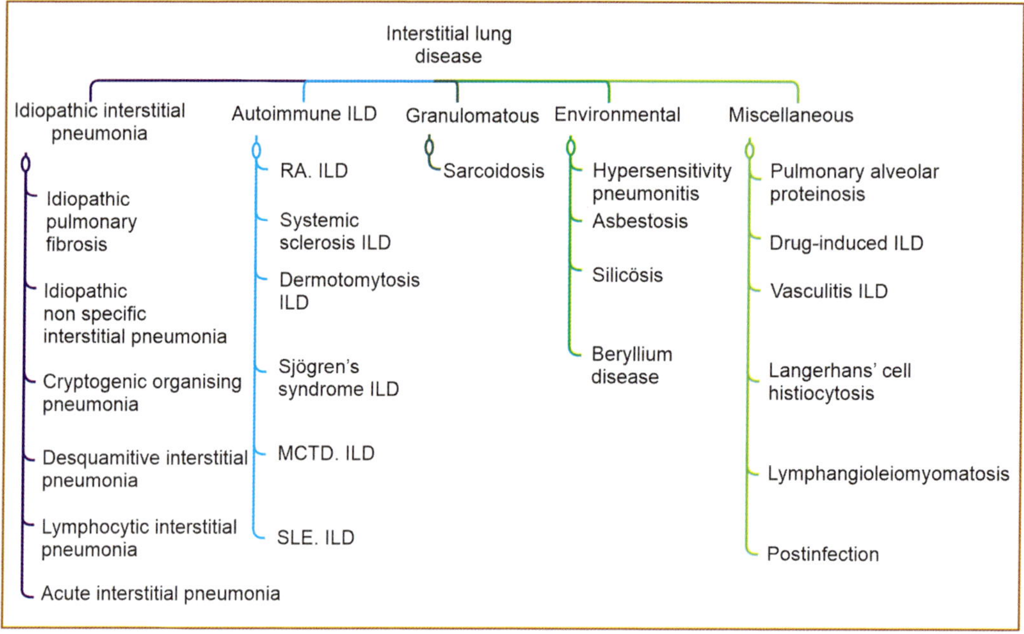

The prognosis of IPF remains poor, with a median survival of 3 years. However, anti-fibrotic therapies such as **pirfenidone** and **nintedanib** have transformed its management, reducing disease progression and improving quality of life.

Hypersensitivity Pneumonitis (HP)

HP results from immune-mediated reactions to inhaled organic antigens. Acute HP presents with fever, cough, and dyspnea, which resolve upon antigen avoidance. Chronic HP is associated with progressive fibrosis, centrilobular nodularity, and ground-glass opacities on HRCT. A bronchoalveolar lavage lymphocytosis (>50%) supports the diagnosis.

Management involves antigen identification and avoidance, with immunosuppressive therapy reserved for fibrotic or progressive disease.

CTD-Associated ILD

Autoimmune diseases, including rheumatoid arthritis (RA), systemic sclerosis (SSc), polymyositis/dermatomyositis, and Sjögren's syndrome, are common causes of ILD. The patterns of fibrosis vary, with UIP commonly seen in RA and non-specific interstitial pneumonia (NSIP) predominating in other CTDs.
- **Systemic sclerosis-associated ILD (SSc-ILD):** Pulmonary involvement occurs in approximately 25% of SSc patients within 3 years of diagnosis. HRCT typically shows NSIP features with ground-glass opacities and coarse reticulations.
  - First-line treatment includes *mycophenolate mofetil* or *cyclophosphamide*, both of which have shown efficacy in improving lung function and quality of life.
- **RA-associated ILD:** Risk factors include smoking, male sex, older age, and high levels of autoantibodies. Management involves corticosteroids and immunosuppressants such as mycophenolate mofetil or rituximab. Methotrexate, despite historical concerns, has not been conclusively linked to ILD development.

Sarcoidosis

Sarcoidosis is a multi-system granulomatous disease of unknown etiology. Pulmonary involvement is common, with HRCT revealing symmetrical hilar lymphadenopathy, perilymphatic nodularity, and upper-zone predominance. Extrapulmonary manifestations include arthritis, uveitis, and cardiac sarcoidosis.

Glucocorticoids remain the mainstay of treatment, with immunosuppressive agents such as methotrexate, leflunomide, and mycophenolate mofetil reserved for refractory cases.

Drug-induced ILD

Certain medications, including **nitrofurantoin**, **bleomycin**, **amiodarone**, and immune checkpoint inhibitors, can cause drug-induced ILD. Management involves discontinuation of the offending drug and initiation of corticosteroids for severe cases.

Emerging Concepts: Progressive Fibrosing ILD

Some ILDs, including IPF, HP, and CTD-ILD, exhibit a progressive fibrosing phenotype characterized by relentless lung function decline and poor prognosis. Advances in anti-fibrotic therapy offer hope for these patients.

Conclusion

Interstitial lung diseases are complex conditions requiring a nuanced approach to diagnosis and management. The integration of advanced imaging techniques, minimally invasive diagnostic modalities, and emerging therapeutic agents has improved outcomes for many patients. However, the prognosis remains poor in several subtypes, highlighting the need for early diagnosis, personalized treatment, and palliative care integration.

FURTHER READING

1. Raghu G, Remy-Jardin M, Myers JL, et al. Diagnosis of Idiopathic Pulmonary Fibrosis. An Official ATS/ERS/JRS/ALAT Clinical Practice Guideline. *Am J Respir Crit Care Med.* 2018;198(5):e44-e68.
2. Tashkin DP, Roth MD, Clements PJ, et al. Mycophenolate mofetil versus oral cyclophosphamide in scleroderma-related interstitial lung disease (SLS II): a randomised controlled trial. *Lancet Respir Med.* 2016;4(9):708–719.

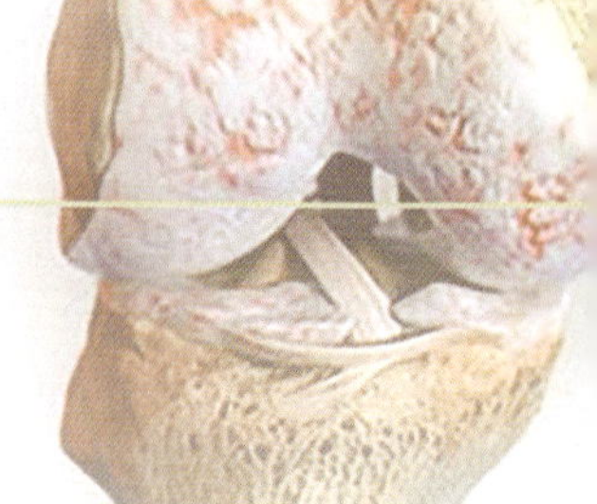

Autoimmune Neuropathy

Spoorthy Kothapalli

Autoimmune neuropathy encompasses a spectrum of conditions in which the body's immune system mistakenly targets components of the peripheral nervous system, leading to inflammation and subsequent nerve damage. When immune-mediated processes affect the blood vessels supplying peripheral nerves, critical ischemia can occur, resulting in nerve damage with potentially profound clinical consequences. This can manifest as chronic, intractable pain, muscle atrophy, impaired functional abilities, and autonomic dysfunction. In some cases, the peripheral nervous system is the sole site of immune attack, a presentation seen in conditions such as nonsystemic autoimmune neuropathy.

Etiopathogenesis

1. Immune mediated demyelination
2. Vasculitis involving vasa vasorum
3. Edema due to inflammation
4. Entrapment due to adjacent synovial inflammation
5. Drugs
6. Amyloidosis
7. Comorbid conditions like diabetes, nutritional deficiency

Clinical Features

About 35–65% of the vasculitic neuropathy patients show the typical clinical picture of a mononeuropathic multiplex where they complain of sudden development of proximal deep aching pain in the limb followed by burning cutaneous pain and focal weakness in the territory of a single nerve and within days to weeks, other nerves become involved. However, half of the patients show other clinical types, mostly painful sensorimotor axonal neuropathy or, rarely, pure sensory neuropathy, mostly with an asymmetric pattern or distal-symmetric neuropathy.

Patients with SVN caused by large nerve arteriole vasculitis frequently develop constitutional symptoms such as weight loss, fatigue, fever, rash, or night sweats. There might be evidence of additional organ involvement, with the presence of hematuria, respiratory symptoms, and abdominal pain, among other features.

Classification

Classification of vasculitis associated with neuropathy (according to Collins et al, 2010).

Primary systemic vasculitis	Secondary systemic vasculitis	Non-systemic or localised vasculitis
Small vessel vasculitis: Microscopic polyangiitis Eosinophilic granulomatosis with polyangiitis Granulomatosis with polyangiitis Essential mixed cryoglobulinemic Henoch–Schönlein purpura	CTD related: Rheumatoid arthritis Systemic lupus erythematosus Sjögren's syndrome Systemic sclerosis Dermatomyositis Mixed connective tissue disease	Diabetic radiculoplexus neuropathy: Diabetic lumbosacral radiculoplexus neuropathy Diabetic cervical radiculoplexus neuropathy Diabetic thoracic radiculopathy Painless diabetic motor neuropathy
Medium vessel vasculitis: Polyarteritis nodosa	Sarcoidosis Behçet's disease Inflammatory bowel disease Hypocomplementemic urticarial vasculitis syndrome	Non-systemic vasculitic neuropathy
Large vessel vasculitis: Giant cell arteritis	Infection (HBV, HCV, HIV, CMV, leprosy, Lyme disease) Drugs Malignancy	Localised cutaneous or neuropathic vasculitis: Cutaneous polyarteritis nodosa

Diagnosis

A good history is important to clinch the diagnosis. Apart from it basic laboratory investigations like Complete blood count, renal function test, liver function test, urinalysis, HbA1c, erythrocyte sedimentation rate, C-reactive protein, antinuclear antibodies, rheumatoid factor, antineutrophil cytoplasmic antibodies, serum protein immunofixation electrophoresis, complement (C3, C4), cryoglobulins, hepatitis B surface antigen, hepatitis C antibodies, and chest X-ray.

Nerve conduction study: Findings that are most supportive of a diagnosis of vasculitic neuropathy are those indicative of asymmetrical or non-length dependent patterns of axonal neuropathy. Sensory nerve action potentials decrease in amplitude and often disappear over the 7–10 days after the ischemic event. The sural and superficial peroneal sensory studies should be compared side-to-side. A 50% interside difference in amplitudes recorded from the same nerve is generally regarded as a meaningful difference.

Nerve biopsy: Most centres choose to biopsy the sural sensory nerve or the superficial peroneal sensory nerve plus peroneus brevis muscle. In upper limb-predominant disorders, the superficial radial nerve is commonly biopsied. It has been suggested that the addition of muscle biopsy improves the yield of definite vasculitis. Large arteriole vasculitic neuropathy typically includes fibrinoid necrosis of the tunica media and intima, but this feature is not characteristic of microvasculitis. In microvasculitis, there is inflammation of the vessel wall with fragmentation and necrosis of the tunica media

The guideline on NSVN from the peripheral nerve society provides diagnostic criteria for probable and definite vasculitic neuropathy. The diagnosis of definite vasculitic neuropathy includes (1) inflammatory cells in the vessel wall accompanied by pathologic evidence of acute or chronic vascular wall damage, and (2) no evidence of another primary disease that mimics vasculitis pathology. Probable vasculitic neuropathy can be suspected, if (1) the criteria for definite vasculitic neuropathy are not completely fulfilled, (2) the neuropathy is predominantly axonal and (3) perivascular inflammation plus signs of vascular damage or pathological predictors of vasculitic neuropathy.

Treatment

The general approach to treatment of SVN is initiation of induction therapy to stop the inflammatory damage, followed by long-term suppression with a maintenance therapy. Maintenance therapy of systemic vasculitis is generally continued for at least 18–24 months after remission is achieved.

High-dose prednisone is standard therapy along with cyclophosphamide is also used for 3–6 months (either pulse or daily oral therapy). For milder symptoms methotrexate can be substituted for cyclophosphamide. Usually recommended starting dose of prednisolone is 1 0 mg/kg per day. In severe cases, intravenous methylprednisolone can be initiated (e.g., 1000 mg intravenous daily for 3–5 days followed by oral daily prednisone). After 1–2 months, tapering can be initiated, with a dose reduction of 5–10 mg every few weeks. Azathioprine or methotrexate should be substituted for cyclophosphamide once remission has been achieved. Second-line maintenance therapies include mycophenolate mofetil, leflunomide, and ciclosporin.

For patients with treatment-refractory disease (unchanged or increased disease activity after 4–6 weeks of cyclophosphamide and corticosteroids or improved but persistent disease activity after 8 weeks of therapy), rituximab is the drug of choice, but other options include IVIg, plasma exchange, mycophenolate mofetil, alemtuzumab, infliximab, antithymocyte globulin, and calcineurin inhibitors.

Drug name	Dose	Side effects
Cyclophosphamide	500–750 mg/m² Per infusion	Bone marrow suppression, hemorrhagic cystitis, serious systemic infections,increased the risk of malignancy (lymphoma, leukemia, transitional cell carcinoma of the bladder, and nonmelanomatous skin cancer)
Methotrexate	15–25 mg/week	Nausea, vomiting, leucopenia, ulcerative stomatitis, fatigue, dizziness, rash, bone marrow suppression, and increased risk of infection, interstitial pneumonitis
Azathioprine	2–3 mg/kg/day	Bone marrow suppression, hepatotoxicity, pancreatitis, and risk of systemic infection.
Rituximab	375 mg/m² intravenous weekly for 4 weeks	hypotension, chills, dyspnea, fever, nausea, vomiting, flushing, angioedema, headache, urticaria, pruritus, pulmonary disease, and infections, including progressive multifocal leukoencephalopathy

FURTHER READING

1. Gwathmey KG, Burns TM, Collins MP, & Dyck PJB (2014). Vasculitic neuropathies. The Lancet Neurology, 13(1),67–82.
2. Collins MP, Dyck PJB, Gronseth GS, et al. Peripheral Nerve Society Guideline on the classification, diagnosis, investigation, and immunosuppressive therapy of non-systemic vasculitic neuropathy: executive summary. J Periph Nerv Syst 2010;15:176–84.

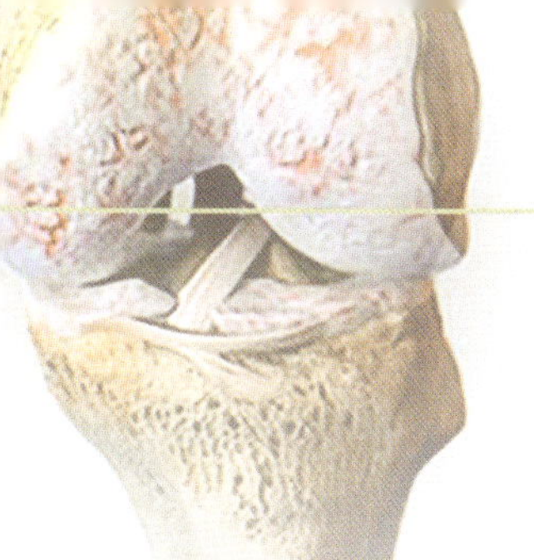

Autoimmune Eye Diseases

Sureja Nayan Patel

INTRODUCTION

Autoimmune eye diseases represent a significant intersection between ophthalmology and rheumatology, as they involve immune-mediated damage to ocular structures. These conditions can lead to severe visual impairment and are often associated with systemic autoimmune diseases. These eye diseases occur when the immune system mistakenly targets ocular tissues, leading to inflammation and damage. Common mechanisms for this aberrant immune response include; **autoantibody production:** Patients may develop autoantibodies against ocular antigens, contributing to tissue damage, **T-cell mediated damage:** Activated T-cells can directly attack ocular tissues or produce cytokines that exacerbate inflammation, and **Molecular mimicry:** Similarities between ocular antigens and microbial antigens can trigger an autoimmune response following an infection.

These processes can be seen in various autoimmune rheumatic diseases, including rheumatoid arthritis (RA), juvenile idiopathic arthritis (JIA), systemic lupus erythematosus (SLE), Sjögren's syndrome (SjS), spondyloarthropathies (SpA), Behcet's disease, sarcoidosis, small vessel vasculitis (ANCA vasculitis), large vessel vasculitis (Takayasu arteritis (TA) and Giant cell arteritis (GCA)) and antiphospholipid syndrome (APS).

Clinical Features

Eye condition	Disease	Symptoms (A) and signs (B)
Dry eyes (Keratoconjunctivitis sicca)	Primary SjS, secondary SjS (RA)	A. Dryness, discomfort, foreign body sensation, corneal ulceration B. Abnormalities on Schirmer's test, eye staining, and tear breakup time (TBUT)
Uveitis	JIA, SpA, Behcet's, sarcoidosis	A. Redness, pain, photophobia, diminished vision, hypopyon B. Cells and flare in the anterior chamber on slit lamp examination. Keratic precipitates (KPs) and hypopyon in few cases.
Episcleritis	RA, ANCA vasculitis	A. Redness and mild or no pain B. Conjunctival congestion

(Contd.)

(Contd.)

Eye condition	Disease	Symptoms (A) and signs (B)
Scleritis	RA, ANCA vasculitis	A. Redness, ocular and periorbital pain B. Conjunctival congestion
Retinal vasculitis	SLE, Behcet's	A. Diminished vision B. Abnormalities on fluorescein angiography and fundoscopy
Optic neuritis	SjS, SLE	A. Diminished vision B. Optic disc edema on fundoscopy
Arteritic anterior/ posterior ischemic optic neuropathy (AAION/ APION)	GCA, SLE	A. Blindness B. Optic disc edema on fundoscopy
Central/branch retinal artery occlusion (CRAO/BRAO)	APS, GCA, TA, SLE	A. Blindness B. Pale retina and cherry red spot on fundoscopy
Central/branch retinal vein occlusion (CRVO/ BRVO)	APS	A. Diminished vision B. Retinal hemorrhages and optic disc edema on fundoscopy
Proptosis due to orbital mass	ANCA vasculitis (Granulomatosis with polyangiitis (GPA), sarcoidosis	A. Diplopia, diminished vision B. Proptosis and orbital mass on imaging

Diagnosis

Accurate diagnosis of autoimmune eye diseases requires a comprehensive assessment that includes:

Patient history: A detailed history focusing on systemic symptoms, previous autoimmune diseases, and family history is crucial.

Ophthalmic examination: Comprehensive eye examinations, including slit-lamp examination, optical coherence tomography (OCT), fluorescein angiography, and visual acuity assessment.

Investigations: Routine investigations like complete blood counts, urine examination, renal and liver function tests should be performed in all the patients. Additionally following investigations needs to be asked for based on the disease suspected.

Suspected disease	Specific investigations
SpA	HLA-B27
SLE	Anti-nuclear antibodies (ANA), complements (C3/C4)
Small vessel vasculitis	Anti-nuclear cytoplasmic antibodies (ANCA)
SjS	ANA, Anti-Ro (SSA), Anti-La (SSB)
APS	Lupus anti-coagulant (LAC), anti-cardiolipin antibodies, anti-beta 2 glycoprotein antibodies
RA	Rheumatoid factor (RF), anti-CCP antibodies
Sarcoidosis	Serum angiotensin convertase enzyme, serum calcium

(Contd.)

(Contd.)

Suspected disease	Specific Investigations
TA/GCA	Magnetic resonance/computed tomography angiography
Behcet's	HLA-B51, Pathergy test
JIA	RF, ANA

Treatment

Based on the type of ocular involvement various treatment options are available which when timely initiated can prevent further complications. Topical drugs like steroids, non-steroidal anti-inflammatory drugs, cyclosporine, lubricants, etc. are usually prescribed by an ophthalmologist. Whereas oral drugs like steroids, sulfasalazine, azathioprine, mycophenolate mofetil, and pilocarpine are given by the rheumatologists. In few cases intravenous cyclophosphamide, and biologics like adalimumab, golimumab, and rituximab are also used depending on the manifestation and the disease.

Prognosis

Most of the autoimmune ocular manifestations when left untreated can lead to complications like corneal ulcers, corneal opacities, keratitis, scleral thinning/perforation, glaucoma, anterior/posterior synechiae, diminished vision, and blindness. Thus, early identification of disease and appropriate treatment can improve the outcomes.

FURTHER READING

1. Kemeny-Beke A, Szodoray P. Ocular manifestations of rheumatic diseases. Int Ophthalmol. 2020;40(2):503–10.
2. Turk MA, Hayworth JL, Nevskaya T, Pope JE. Ocular Manifestations in Rheumatoid Arthritis, Connective Tissue Disease, and Vasculitis: A Systematic Review and Metaanalysis. J Rheumatol. 2021;48(1):25–34.
3. Hochberg Textbook of Rheumatology.

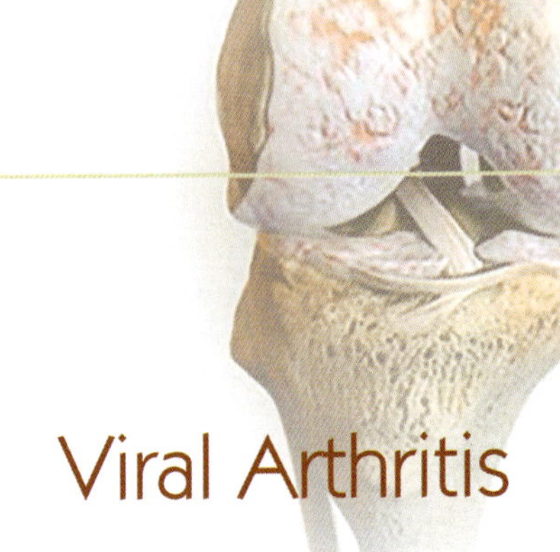

Viral Arthritis

Pothireddy Mohit Kumar Reddy, Sarath Chandra Mouli Veeravalli

INTRODUCTION

Viral arthritis is inflammation of the joints caused by viral infections, accounting for about 1% of acute arthritis cases. While chronic viruses like hepatitis B and C have become less prominent due to vaccinations and antiviral therapies, other viruses such as Zika, chikungunya, dengue, and SARS-CoV-2 are increasingly significant. Diagnosis depends on clinical features, epidemiological data, and serological testing. Most cases are self-limiting, but some may require specific antiviral treatments. A thorough understanding of the evolving viral landscape is essential for effective diagnosis and management of viral arthritis.

Clinical Features

Viral arthritis typically occurs during the viral prodrome, featuring sudden-onset polyarthritis that may mimic RA (symmetrical small joint involvement), preceded by fever, and sometimes associated with other symptoms like icterus in viral hepatitis. A thorough history of exposures and travel should be considered.

A summary of viral infections and their features is detailed in Table 24.1.

Diagnosis

Most cases of viral arthritis can be diagnosed clinically, but serological testing can identify specific etiologies that may impact treatment such as HIV, hepatitis, rubella, mumps, varicella, dengue, and chikungunya. Testing also helps in assessing disease patterns and extra-articular symptoms. A positive IgM or a fourfold increase in IgG titers indicates recent infection. Radiologic findings usually show non-erosive changes, primarily soft-tissue swelling, depending on the specific viral condition.

Treatment

Viral arthritis is usually mild, self limiting requiring only symptomatic treatment with analgesics or NSAIDs, and occasionally low-dose steroids. Chronic chikungunya arthritis resembles RA, characterized by persistent arthralgia and an inflammatory response. Treatments like hydroxychloroquine and other DMARDs (methotrexate, sulfasalazine, leflunomide) have been evaluated, but studies yield inconsistent results. Currently,

Table 24.1: Clinical presentation of viral arthritis

Virus	Typical presenting features	Characteristics of arthritis	Likelihood of presenting with arthritis	Duration of arthritis	Comments
EBV	Pharyngitis, cervical lymphadenopathy, fever	Arthralgia > Arthritis	Very low	Days	Often have myalgias with acute infection
Herpes viruses	CMV—infectious mononucleosis. VZV—chickenpox/shingles HSV—mucosal infections	CMV—swollen Knees—noninflammatory. VZV—MC knee HSV—MC knee	Very low	Days	Rarely associated with arthritis; specific treatment for some non-articular manifestations
Adenovirus and Enterovirus	Upper respiratory tract infections, GI symptoms, conjunctivitis	Predominantly knees.	Very low	Days	
Parvovirus B19	Children—viral exanthem common than arthritis. Adults—arthralgia >arthritis, F>M.	Children—large joint Oligoarticular, adults-RA-like pattern (small joints in additive nature)	High	Days to months	Recurrence also reported
Hepatitis A	Flu-like illness followed by jaundice. Arthralgia—0–14%.	MC—Knee and ankle arthralgias	Low	Days	Arthralgia > arthritis No chronicity
Hepatitis B	Malaise, rash, jaundice. Arthritis—F>M. MC in young adults.	Arthritis—RA like distribution preceding icteric phase, can be migratory	Moderate	Days/weeks	No chronicity Non-erosive

(Contd.)

(Contd.)

Virus	Typical presenting features	Characteristics of arthritis	Likelihood of presenting with arthritis	Duration of arthritis	Comments
Hepatitis C	Malaise, jaundice arthralgia as part of mixed cryoglobulinemia	Arthritis—unusual.	Moderate	Weeks, months	Chronic arthralgia (20%).
HIV	Acute infection—infectious Mononucleosis—like illness at seroconversion in some patients. Chronic HIV—painful articular syndrome (disproportionate pain) HIV associated arthritis—at any stage	Acute infection—knees asymmetric arthritis Chronic HIV—asymmetric severe arthralgias, lower limb predominant. No arthritis	Low	Acute—weeks Chronic—self limiting in 24 hrs.	Arthritis, arthralgia with acute infection. Increased incidence of several rheumatic diseases in chronic infection
Alpha viruses (7 viruses associated with viral arthritis)	CHIKV—arthralgia, myalgia, fever, rash (several days after the onset of joint symptoms, short-lived, involving—face (nose) "Chick sign", trunk, and flexor surfaces of the extremities). F>M	Symmetrical. MC joints—digits, wrists, knees and ankles. Chronic arthritis relapsing and remitting in 60–80% of patients and unremitting in 20–40%.	Very high	Weeks to months	Can rarely be associated with neurological complications like encephalitis, GBS, optic neuritis.

(Contd.)

(Contd.)

Virus	Typical presenting features	Characteristics of arthritis	Likelihood of presenting with arthritis	Duration of arthritis	Comments
Flavivirus	Dengue—arthralgias, rash, leucopenia, thrombocytopenia, transaminitis	True arthritis, synovitis rare	Moderate	Days to weeks	Lethal forms can present like DHF,DSS
Mumps	Parotitis and lymphadenopathy,	Migratory arthralgias involving both large and small joints	Very low	Weeks	No joint damage
Rubella	Acute maculopapular rash, sparing the palms and soles. Arthralgia >arthritis.	Symmetric,migratory or additive. MC—small joints of hands, wrists, knee	High	Weeks	Can occur with rubella vaccine also.

CHIKV: Chikungunya; HBV: Hepatitis B virus; HCV: Hepatitis C virus; RA: Rheumatoid Arthritis; MC: Most common; FM: Female; M: Male; DHF: Dengue hemorrhagic fever; DSS: Dengue shock syndrome

methotrexate, with or without other DMARDs and steroids, is the standard treatment for chronic chikungunya arthritis. For patients who do not respond to these therapies, biologics (TNF i) may be considered. Other viral infections like HIV, hepatitis will require specific antiviral therapy.

Clinical Snippet

A 34-year-old woman presented with a fever that later subsided, but she subsequently developed polyarthritis affecting the bilateral small joints of her hands and both feet. Chikungunya PCR testing confirmed the diagnosis. She was initially treated with NSAIDs for the first week; however, she continued to experience persistent joint pain and synovitis in both wrists and ankles. Due to the ineffectiveness of the NSAIDs, she was prescribed a short course of oral steroids along with hydroxychloroquine, and the steroids were gradually tapered over a brief period.

Prognosis

Most viral arthritis cases are self-limited and result in no residual joint damage. However, chronic arthritis like chikungunya may need long term therapies due to potential joint damage and significant morbidity.

FURTHER READING

1. Viral arthritis. In: Textbook of Rheumatology, Firestein & Kelley
2. Marks M, Marks JL. Viral arthritis. Clin Med (Lond). 2016.
3. National guidelines for clinical management of chikungunya virus 2023.

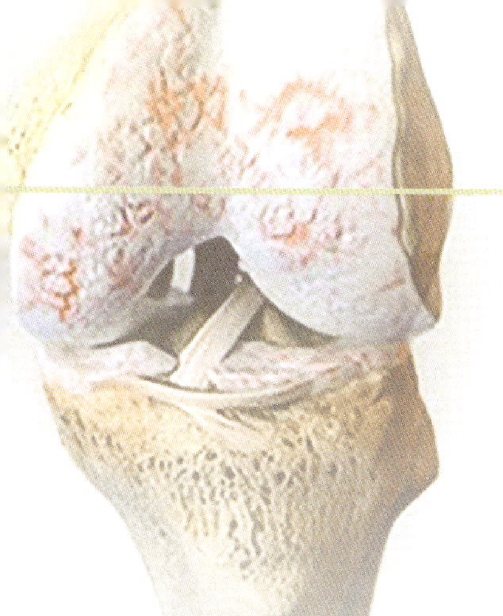

Crystal Arthropathies

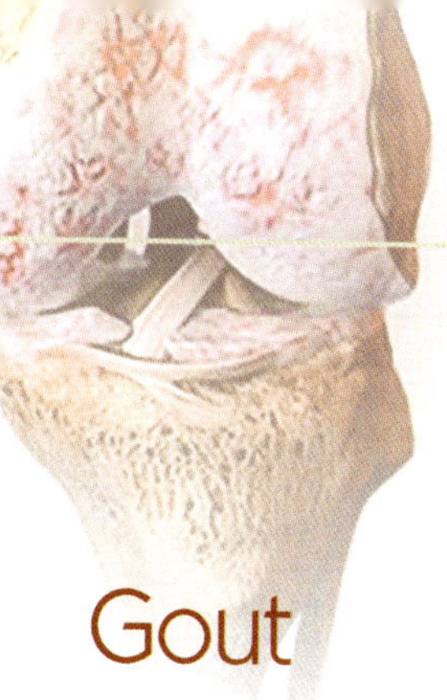

Gout

Sneha Babu, Hema M

Gout is a chronic inflammatory disorder characterised by the deposition of monosodium urate (MSU) crystals in articular tissues. It typically affects one or more joints, most commonly the first metatarsophalangeal joint in the lower limbs.

Risk Factors

Modifiable: Hypertension, obesity, hyperlipidemia, diabetes, cardiovascular diseases, alcohol consumption, chronic kidney disease, and dietary factors (red meat, seafood, organ meats). Certain drugs (e.g., diuretics, low-dose aspirin, ethambutol, pyrazinamide, cyclosporine) can also affect urate levels.

Non-modifiable: Age 40–60, genetic variants, male gender, and ethnicity.

Pathogenesis

Uric Acid Metabolism

Uric acid is the final product of purine metabolism and balance between its production and excretion is essential to maintain normal serum uric acid concentration.

Normal Uric Acid Levels

Men: 3.4–7.0 mg/dl
Women: 2.4–6.0 mg/dl

High uric acid levels (hyperuricemia > 6.8 mg/dl): May cause gout and are linked to kidney stones and renal issues.

Low uric acid levels: Less common, but may indicate conditions such as liver disease or certain genetic disorders.

Uric Acid Production

Purines (guanosine [GMP], inosine [IMP]) are metabolised into uric acid by xanthine oxidase. Salvage pathways involving HGPRTase and APRTase convert purine metabolites back to IMP/GMP.

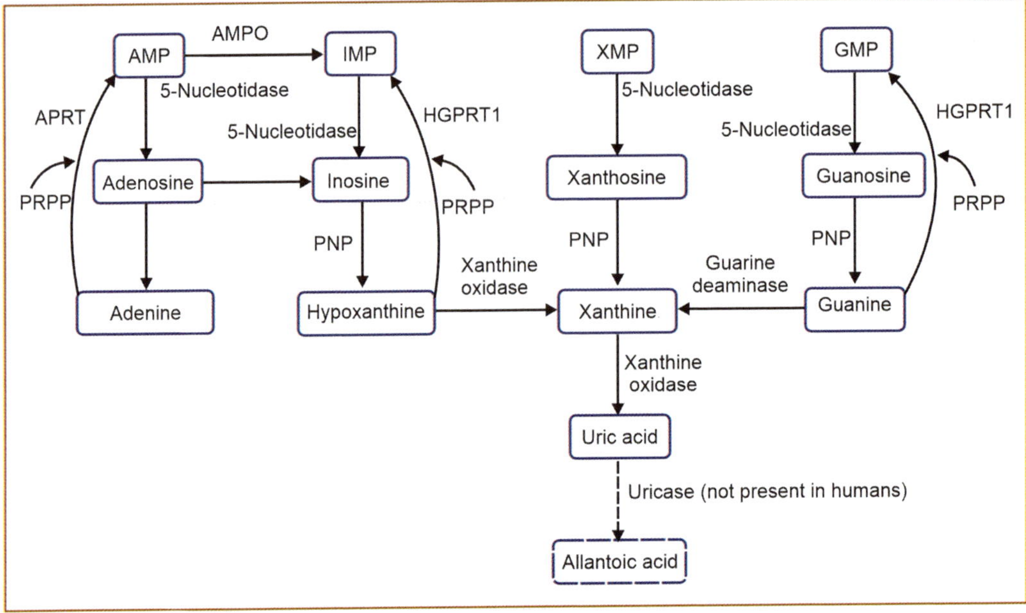

Uric Acid Excretion

Uric acid is primarily excreted through the kidneys (two-thirds) and the gastrointestinal tract (one-third). Renal excretion involves ultrafiltration, reabsorption (URAT1, OAT4, OAT10, GLUT 9), and secretion (OAT1, OAT2, OAT3, ABCG2, NPT1, NPT4, and MRP4)

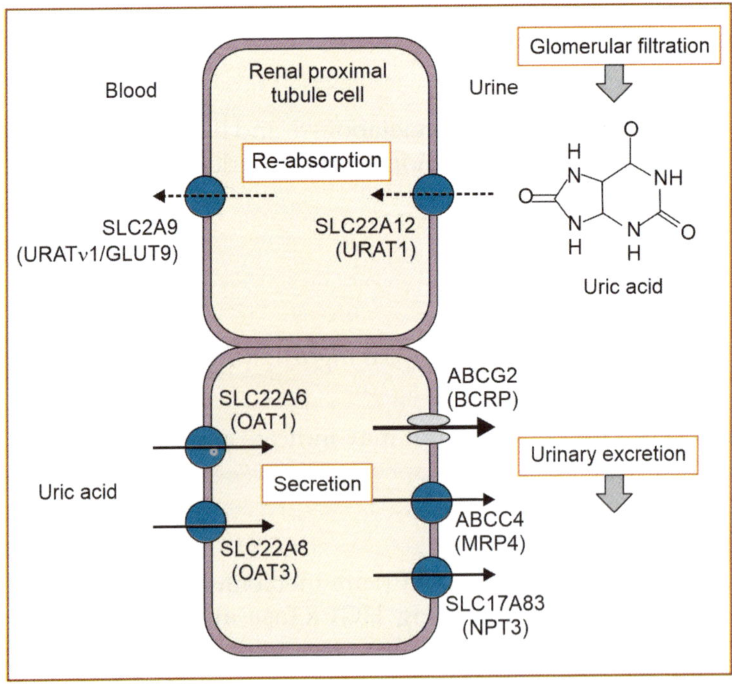

Hyperuricemia and Gout

Gout is driven by elevated uric acid from overproduction or under-excretion.

Overproduction arises from increased purine synthesis, PRPP synthase overactivity, salvage pathway defects (e.g., Lesch-Nyhan, Kelley-Seegmiller syndrome) or increased cell turnover (e.g., leukemia, lymphoma).

Under-excretion occurs from impaired renal function, chronic kidney disease, or medications.

Crystal Formation

The sine qua non of acute gout is the precipitation of uric acid.

When uric acid levels exceed 6.8 mg/dl, it crystallizes into needle-shaped MSU crystals that deposit in tissues, especially joints.

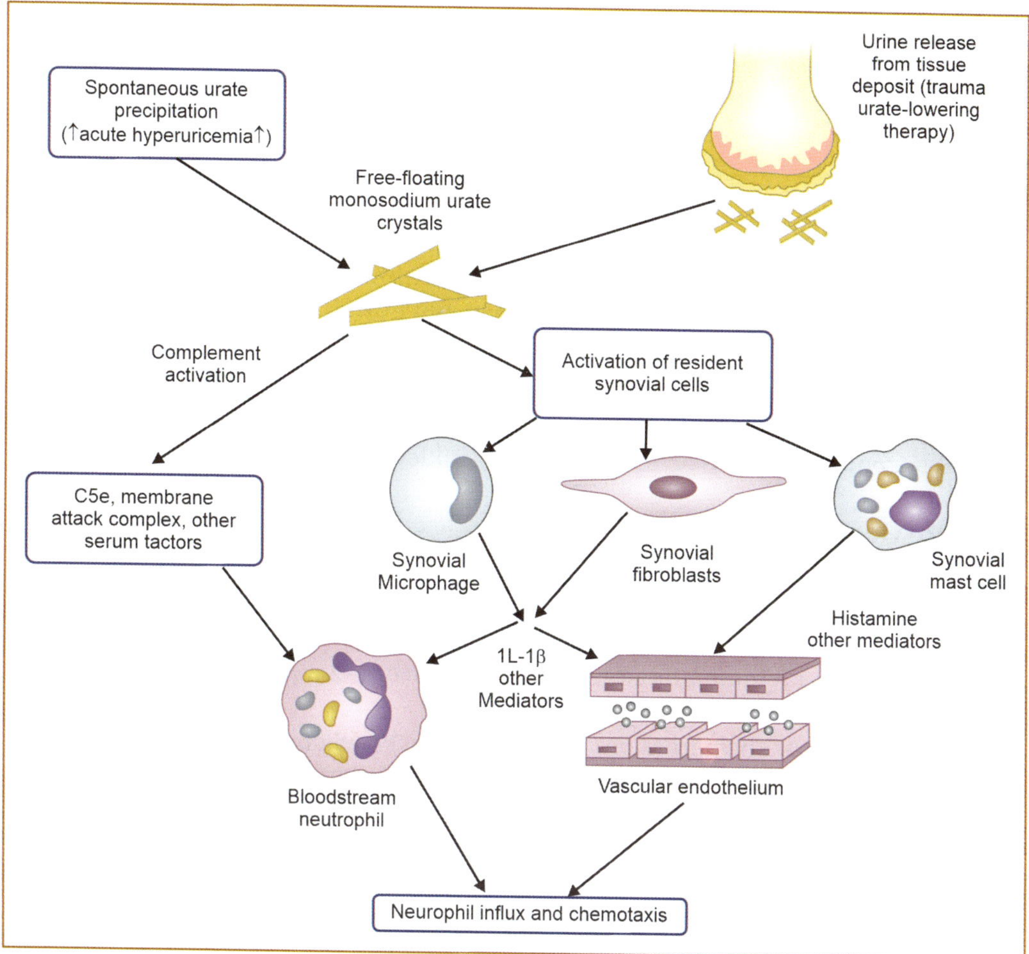

Inflammatory Response

Urate crystal activates synovial macrophages and fibroblasts, triggering inflammation, complement and NLRP3 inflammasome activation. This releases pro-inflammatory cytokines (e.g., IL-1, TNF, IL-6), causing strong inflammation. Repeated deposition can cause chronic joint damage.

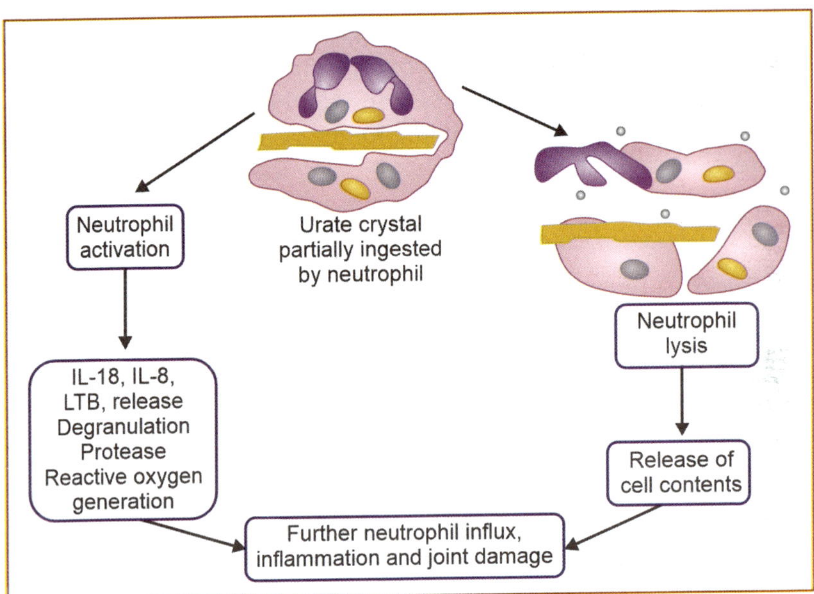

Gout pathogenesis involves interplay between uric acid metabolism, crystal formation, and inflammation, influenced by genetic and environmental factors. Large genome-wide association studies (GWAS) have identified key genetic variants, mainly in genes encoding urate transporters in kidney and gut.

Clinical Features of Gout

Gout typically presents as acute monoarthritis, often affecting first metatarsophalangeal joint. Less commonly, it involves the midfoot, ankle and knee.

Stages of Gout

- **Asymptomatic hyperuricemia:** Elevated uric acid levels in the blood without symptoms that can last for years.
- **Acute gout attack:** Characterized by joint inflammation—pain, redness, swelling, and warmth peaking within 24 hours and resolving over 1–2 weeks. Systemic symptoms may also occur.
- **Intercritical gout:** The period between acute attacks when flare symptoms subside. Even during the asymptomatic phase, chronic inflammation may persist with continuous macrophage activity.
- **Chronic tophaceous gout:** Chronic untreated gout thus leads to tophi, macroscopic monosodium urate deposits. Tophi appear as non-tender, chalk like nodules under transparent skin with vascularity, typically found in joints, tendons (Achilles), ears, olecranon bursae, finger pads. Compressive neuropathies like carpal tunnel syndrome can develop.

Long Term Complications

High monosodium urate levels drive inflammation, oxidative stress and endothelial dysfunction, leading to atherosclerosis, cardiovascular and chronic kidney diseases.

Investigations

The gold standard for diagnosis is arthrocentesis, identifying MSU crystals as negatively birefringent needle-shaped crystals under a polarizing microscope. Blood tests reveal hyperuricemia (>6.8 mg/dl) or normal levels. ESR and CRP may be elevated during acute attacks. Measuring 24-hour urinary uric acid excretion is also valuable.

Imaging

Non-invasive techniques are increasingly used, revealing key findings like the double contour and snowstorm sign, and occasionally intratendinous tophi. X-ray may show bony erosions and joint space narrowing, while MRI helps assess complications like tendon rupture, spinal involvement or infection. Marrow edema on MRI suggests osteomyelitis. Dual energy CT (DECT) is also a useful tool.

Treatment

For acute flares, corticosteroids, NSAIDS, colchicine are commonly used, alongside rest, ice, limb elevation and hydration. Urate lowering therapy—xanthine oxidase inhibitors, uricosuric agents are initiated after the flare resolves.

Medication	Type	Typical Dosage
Colchicine	Anti-inflammatory	1.2 mg initially, then 0.6 mg after 1 hour (max 1.8 mg/day)
Indomethacin	NSAID	25 mg two times daily until pain subsides
Naproxen	NSAID	250 mg twice daily
Prednisone	Corticosteroid	30–40 mg/day for 5–10 day, then taper
Allopurinol	Xanthine oxidase inhibitor	100–300 mg/day (start at 100 mg, increase gradually)
Febuxostat	Xanthine oxidase inhibitor	40–80 mg/day
Probenecid	Uricosuric agent	500 mg twice daily (may increase)
lesinurad	Uricosuric agent	200 mg/day in combination therapy

Anti IL-1 agents like Canakinumab are also used. Novel drugs like arhalofenate, PPAR gamma ligand and verinurad, which promote uric acid excretion via URAT 1 inhibition, are under trial.

Dietary/Lifestyle Interventions

Limitation of purine-rich meat and seafood, avoiding alcohol and sweetened drinks, increased low-fat dairy intake, and weight reduction are advised.

Clinical Vignette

A 55-year-old male patient presents with sudden, sharp, and severe pain in his right big toe and ankle, worsening at night. The toe is swollen, red, and warm. He has history of diabetes, hypertension, alcohol use, and non-vegetarian diet. He reports similar symptoms over the past 9 months. On examination, there is tenderness, warmth, erythema over the metatarsophalangeal joint and ankle with restriction of movements. Blood investigations revealed increased uric acid, ESR and CRP levels.

This patient was treated with oral colchicine. He was later started on tablet febuxostat 40 mg once daily.

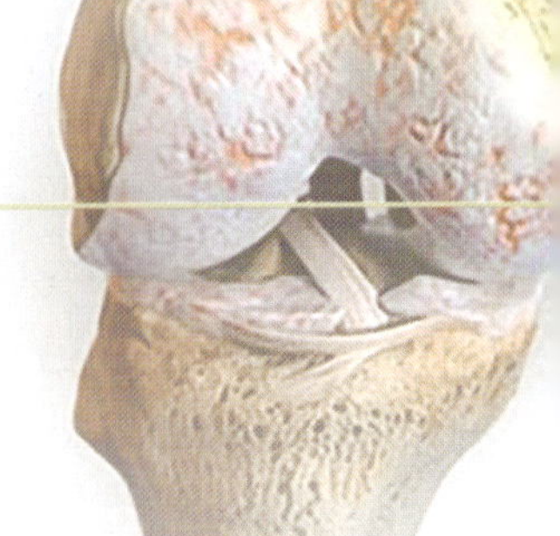

Calcium Pyrophosphate Disease

Manisha Ashwin Daware

INTRODUCTION

Calcium pyrophosphate deposition (CPPD) disease is a type of crystal arthropathy characterised by the pathological deposition of calcium pyrophosphate (CPP) crystals inside joints. For clinical purposes, the term CPPD means the deposition of CPP crystals and CPPD disease refers to symptomatic presentations of the same.

The exact pathophysiology of CPPD is unknown, but it is considered an immune response to the deposition of calcium pyrophosphate (CPP) crystals in joints. Mechanisms of the inflammatory response include the activation of the NLRP3 inflammasome, like gout.

The clinical presentation of CPPD disease mimics other inflammatory arthritis like gout, rheumatoid arthritis, polymyalgia rheumatica, or non-inflammatory conditions like osteoarthritis; which can potentially delay diagnosing CPPD.

There is no known treatment to dissolve CPPD crystals, hence, the treatment target we use in clinical practice is mainly the control of local inflammation.

Clinical Features

The prevalence of CPPD disease increases with ageing. The exact prevalence is unknown as many cases are asymptomatic and are incidentally diagnosed on routine radiographs. It is rarely seen under the age of 55, but occurs in 10–15% of people between the ages of 65 and 75 years and in 30–60% of those over 85.

There is no gender difference: CPPD has been noted to affect men and women equally.

The prevalence of CPPD changes depending on the type of cartilage affected. At least in older populations (>80 years of age), the involvement is found to be 23.3% for hyaline cartilage and 46.7% for fibrocartilage.[5]

Knees and wrists are the most frequently involved peripheral joints on imaging and are most often symptomatic, followed by shoulders, acromioclavicular joints, hips, knees, ankles, and feet.

Clinical Phenotype

1. **Asymptomatic:** Diagnosed on radiographs done for other purpose
2. **Acute inflammation:** Can be mono, oligoarticular, or polyarticular (pseudogout) or crowned dens syndrome.

3. **Chronic inflammatory arthritis:** Chronic mono, oligo, polyarthritis (psuedo-rheumatoid arthritis)
4. CPPD and osteoarthritis

Risk Factors for CPPD

1. Ageing is the most common risk factor for CPPD,
2. Local joint injury to the joint
3. Inherited and acquired metabolic diseases (primary hyperparathyroidism, hereditary hemochromatosis, hypomagnesemia, familial hypocalciuric hypocalcemia, and hypophosphatasia)
4. ANKH (inorganic pyrophosphate transport regulator) gene and the osteoprotegerin gene mutation—Premature and severe presentation.

Unlike primary osteoarthritis, sex and BMI do not seem to be risk factors for CPPD[7].

Diagnosis

Diagnosis of CPPD needs a compatible, clinical presentation and the identification of CPP crystals in the synovial fluids by polarised-light microscopy or typical imaging evidence of CPP crystal deposition. Till now, radiographic, articular chondrocalcinosis has been used as a surrogate for CPPD.

In 2023, the American College of Rheumatology (ACR) and EULAR developed classification criteria for CPPD disease[8] (Table 26.1), the development of new classification criteria will result in an advancement in clinical research for this disease.

The 2023 ACR–EULAR classification criteria for CPPD disease considers:
1. Risk factors (i.e., age, metabolic or inherited risk factors, and hand osteoarthritis),
2. Clinical presentations (i.e., crowned dens syndrome or pattern of inflammatory arthritis), and
3. Findings from synovial fluid examination and imaging (i.e., presence or absence of chondrocalcinosis in symptomatic joints and the number of joints affected) to classify a patient as having CPPD disease.

Treatment

Medications like non-steroidal anti-inflammatory drugs (NSAIDs), colchicine, and low-dose steroids are used to control acute inflammation. In case of no response or chronic presentation, the long-term use of colchicine; hydroxychloroquine; or low dose, weekly methotrexate has been used.

Table 26.2 highlights different medications used for the treatment of CPPD.

Prognosis

As evidenced by data obtained from various studies, there is a substantial variation in the outcomes reported in CPPD. Outcomes that map to imaging manifestations, joint pain and response to treatment domains are most often reported. There are very few studies mapped to domains related to life impact, longevity or societal/resource use. The core domain to study CPPD outcome needs further evaluation.

Table 26.1: 2023 classification criteria for CPPD

Definition of criteria

The CPPD disease classification criteria should be applied in the following order:

1. **Entery criterion:** Ever had at laest one episode of joint pain, swelling or tenderness.[1]
2. **Absolute exculsion criteria:** All symptoms are more likely explained by an alternative condition (such as rheumatoid arthritis, gout, psoriatic arthritis, OA, etc.)
3. **Sufficient criteria:** Presence of either crowned dens syndrome or synovial fluid analysis demonstrating CPP crystals in a joint with swelling, tenderness, or pain.[2]

An individual is classifieds as having CPPD disease if the entry criterion is met, exclusion criteria are not met, and at leastone sufficient criterion is fulfilled. If none of the sufficient criteria are present, an individual is classified as having CPPD disease if the sum of the criteria is >56 points.

Scoring of criteria

Items can be scorved if they were ever present during a patient's lifetime. If a patient fulfills >1 item in a given domain, only the highest weighted item will be scored. Imaging of a least one symptomatic joint by CR, US, CT, or DECT is required.

Domains and levels	Points
A. Age at onset of joint symptoms (pain, swelling, and/or tendemess)	
≤60 years	0
>60 years	4
B. Time course and symptoms of inflammatory artheritis[3]	
No persistent or typical inflammatory arthritis	0
Persistent inflammatory arthritis	9
One typical acute arthritis episode	12
More than one typical acute arthritis episode	16
C. Sites of typical episode(s) of inflammatory arthritis in peripheral joints	
First MTP joint	–6
No typical episode(s)	0
Joint(s) other thant wrist, knee, or first MTP joint	5
Wrist	8
Knee	9
D. Related metabolic diseases[4]	
None	
Present	

(Contd.)

(*Contd.*)

E. Synovial fluid crystal analysis from a symptomatic joint[5]	
CPP crystals absent on ≥2 occasions	−7
CPP crystals absent on 1 occasion	−1
Not performed	0
F. OA of hand/wrist on imaging (defined as present if the K/L score is ≥2)	
None of the below findings or no wrist/hand imaging performed	0
OA of radiocarpal hoints bilaterally	2
≥2 of the following findings: STT joint OA without first CMC joint OA; second MCP joint OA; third MCP joint OA	7
G. Imaging evidence of CPPD in symptomatic peripherial joint(s)[6]	
None on US, CT, or DECT (and absent on CR or CR not performed)	−4
None on CR (and US, CT, DECT not performed)	0
Present on either CR, US, CT, or DECT	16
H. Number of peripheral joints with evidence of CPPD on any imaging modality regardless of symptoms[6]	
None	0
1	16
2–3	23
≥4	25

CR: Conventional radiography; US: Ultrasound; MTP: Metatarsophalangeal; K/L: Kellgren/Lawrence; STT: Scaphotrapeziotrapezoid; CMC: Carpometacarpal; MCP: Metacarpophalangeal.

[1]Episode occuring in a peripheral joint or, in the case of crowned dens syndrome, an axial joint such as C1/C2.

[2]Crowned dens syndrome is defined as presence of (a) clinical features and (b) imaging features. Clinical include acute or subacute onset of severe pain localized to the upper neck with elevated inflammation markers, limited rotation, and often fever. Mimicking conditions such as polymyalgia rheumatica and meningitis should be excluded. Imagaing features include conventional computed tomography (CT) showing calcific deposits, typically linear and less dense thatn cortical bone, in the transverse retro-odontoid ligament (transverse ligament of the atlas), often with an appearance of 2 parallel lines in axial views. Calcifications at the atlanto-axial joint, alar ligament, and/or in pannus adjacement to the tip of the dens are also characteristic Dual-energy computed tomography (DECT) features include a dual-energy index between 0.016 and 0.036. Both the clinical features and the imaging features must be present. Sufficient criteria are also met if calcium pyrophosphate (CPP) crytals are demonstrated on his-topathologic analysis of the joint tissue, provided that the patient is eligible for classification, i.e., does not already meet the exclusion criteria. For instance, articualr cartilage CPP crystal deposition in patients with end-stage osteoarthritis (OA) cannot be sued to classify the patient as having calcium pyrophosphate deposition (CPPD) disease when *all* symptoms are better explainrf by the presence of OA (exdusion criteria).

[3]Persistent inflammatory arthritis was defined as ongoing joint swelling with pain and/or warmth in ≥1 joint(s). Typical episode was defined as an episode with acute onset or acute worsening of joint pain with swelling and /or warmth that resolves irrespective of treatment.

[4]Indluding hereditary hemochromatosis, primary hyperparathyroidism, hypomagnesemia, Gitelman syndrome, hypophosphatasis, or familial history of CPPD disease.

[5]Synovial fluid analysis should be performed by anindividual trained in the use of compensated polarized light microsocopy for crystal identification.

[6]Imaging of at least one symptomatic peripheral joint by CR, US, CT, or DECT is required to be considered for classification if sufficient criteria are not met. Imaging evidence of CPPD refers to calcification of the fibrocartilage or hyaline cartilage. Do not score calcification of the synovial membrane, joint capsule, or tendon. Imaging definitions are published elsewhere (21). Only consider involvement of peripheral joints.

Table 26.2: Medications used for treatment of CPPD

Drug group	Drug name	Dose	Toxicity/Contraindication	Special notes
NSAIDs	Aceclofenac/ Naproxen/ Etoricoxib	Depends on drug used	Depends on drug used	Avoid in renal and liver disease, and hypersensitivity
Colchicine	Colchicine	For prevention: 0.6 to 1.2 mg daily in one or two doses. (Maximum dose is 1.2 mg/day.) acute attacks 1.2 mg at the first sign of a flare followed by 0.6 mg an hour later.	Diarrhea	Should be avoided in combination with CYP3A4 inhibitors (many antifungals, antivirals, and P-glycoprotein inhibitors like cyclosporine, ranolazine
Corticosteroids	Prednisolone/ Methylprednisone/ Deflazacort	Prednisolone equivalent dose 0.5–1 mg/kg (depending on severity of inflammation	BP rise, weight gain, cushingoid features, hyperglycemia	Can be used in oral or intra-articular form. Long term use should be avoided
Hydroxychloroquine		200–400 mg per day	Skin rashes, maculopathy	Renal impairment needs dose adjustment
Methotrexate		10–15 mg/ week	Nausea, vomiting, mucositis, bone marrow suppression	Avoid in liver disease, severe kidney failure
IL 1 inhibitor	Anakinra	100 mg OD for 3 days	Injection site reaction, hypersensitivity	Data is mostly extrapolated from gout treatment
		100 mg OD for 3 days	Injection site reaction, hypersensitivity	At present, not available in India

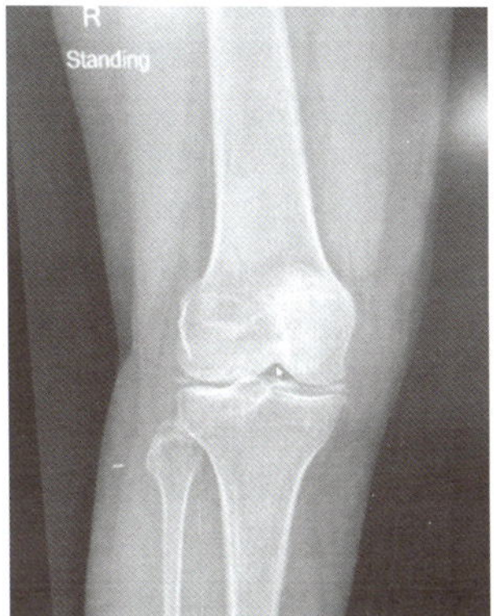

Fig. 26.1: Chondrocalcinosis of both medial and lateral menisci of right knee

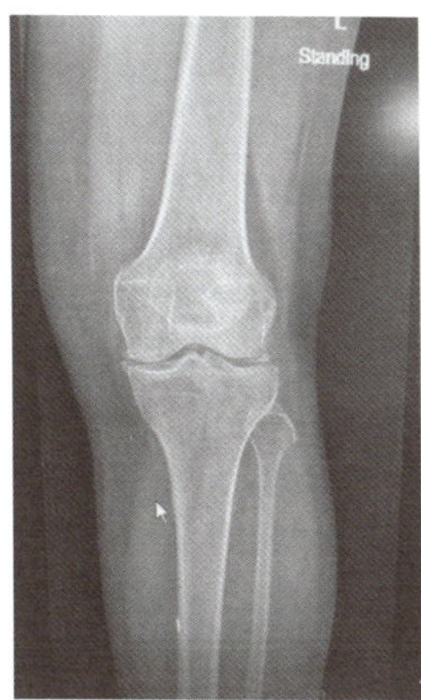

Fig. 26.2: Linear calcification of medial and lateral menisci of left knee

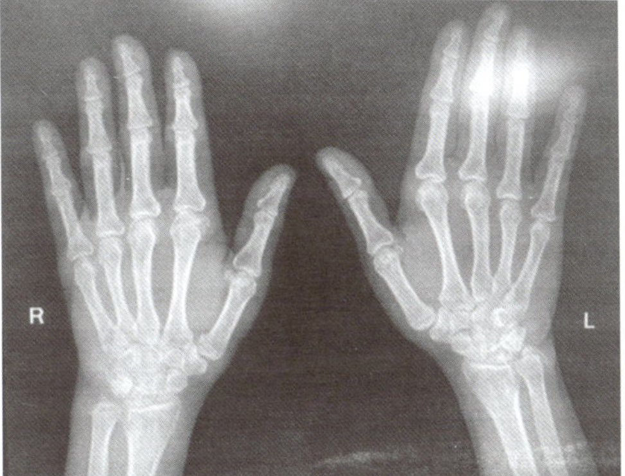

Fig. 26.3: Chondrocalcinosis of triangular cartilage of bilateral wrists

Clinical Snippet

A 55-year-old female came with a history of chronic onset inflammatory arthritis involving bilateral small joints of hands, and wrists. Laboratory investigations showed high inflammatory markers (ESR and CRP), negative rheumatoid factor, and negative anti-CCP antibody assays. Her X-ray hands revealed bilateral triangular fibrocartilage calcification with ulnar styloid erosion and chondrocalcinosis of her second MCP joints, suggestive of CPPD disease. X-ray Knees also revealed chondrocalcinosis (Figs 26.1 to 26.3). She was managed with NSAIDs and oral steroids in tapering doses with partial response, and then was also put on oral methotrexate in a dose of 15 mg/week. She has shown good symptom relief with this combination.

FURTHER READING

1. Zhang W, Doherty M, Bardin T, et al. European league against rheumatism recommendations for calcium pyrophosphate deposition. Part 1: terminology and diagnosis. Ann Rheum Dis 2011;70: 563–70.
2. Adinolfi A, Sirotti S, Sakellariou G, et al. Which are the most frequently involved peripheral joints in calcium pyrophosphate crystal deposition at imaging? A systematic literature review and meta-analysis by the OMERACT ultrasound—CPPD subgroup. Front Med (Lausanne) 2023; 10: 1131362.
3. Abhishek A, Tedeschi SK, Pascart T, et al. The 2023 ACR/EULAR classification criteria for calcium pyrophosphate deposition disease. Arthritis Rheumatol 2023;75:1703–13.

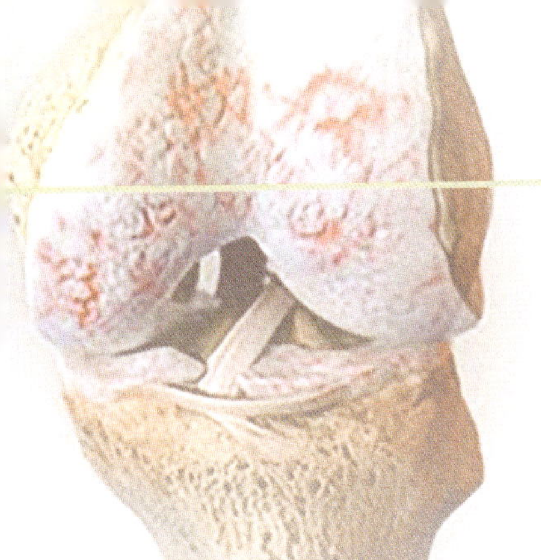

Degenerative and Metabolic Diseases

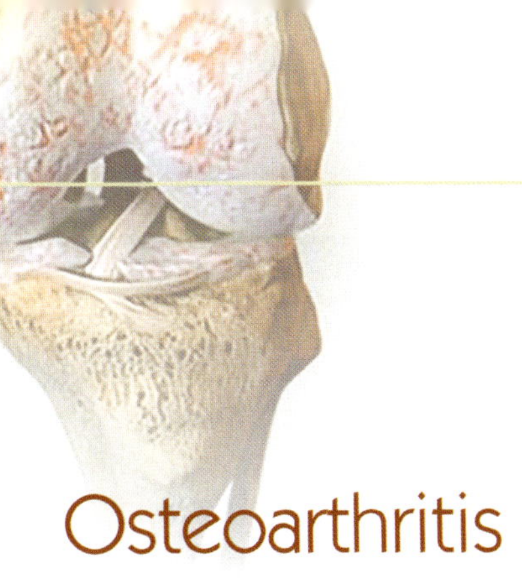

Osteoarthritis

Shweta Agarwal

INTRODUCTION

Osteoarthritis (OA) is the most common arthritis of the global population. It was considered an age-related degenerative disease affecting articular cartilage, particularly weight-bearing joints. However, increasing evidence on synovial inflammation is now available. Different biomechanical factors lead to the activation of inflammatory cytokines like IL-1, IL-6 and TNF which induce the production of inflammatory mediators. These mediators escalate the catabolic pathways and cellular apoptosis and inhibit repair. Various risk factors for developing OA are given in Box 27.1.

OA can be primary (no identifiable aetiology) or secondary (underlying aetiology), although both are similar pathologically. Common causes of secondary OA are enumerated in Box 27.2.

Clinical Features

Primary OA involves knees, hand interphalangeal, 1st carpometacarpal, spine and hips most commonly, though shoulder and temporomandibular joints can also be affected. Usual symptoms and signs of OA have been tabulated in Table 27.1.

Diagnosis

OA is usually diagnosed clinically and/or radiographically. Laboratory examination may be needed occasionally to differentiate from alternative etiologies. Synovial fluid

Box 27.1: Risk factors for OA
Age
Female gender
Genetic predisposition
Obesity
Type of joint
Joint malalignment
Trauma to the joint
Presence of inflammatory arthritis

Box 27.2: Causes of secondary OA
Metabolic disorders—calcium crystal deposition, hemochromatosis, acromegaly
Local factors—limb length discrepancy, congenital dislocation, hypermobility syndromes, epiphyseal dysplasias
Trauma/surgery
Inflammatory arthritis—rheumatoid arthritis, septic arthritis
Charcot joint

Table 27.1: Clinical features of OA

Symptoms	*Signs*
Pain	Crepitus
Early morning stiffness <30 min	Restricted range of motion
'Gelling'–stiffness after inactivity	Deformities
Bony enlargement	Heberden's (DIP) and Bouchard's (PIP) nodes
Sounds from joint	Joint line tenderness
Swelling of joint	Surrounding bursitis
Limitation of movement	Swelling of joint

may reveal calcium pyrophosphate crystals in a substantial number of patients though the rest of the parameters are usually normal or in favour of mild inflammation at most. American College of Rheumatology (ACR) gave classification criteria for knee, hand and hip OA (Box 27.3) based on clinical and radiographic features.

Box 27.3: ACR radiologic and clinical criteria for osteoarthritis

Knee: Clinical
1. Knee pain for most days of prior month
2. Crepitus with active joint motion
3. Morning stiffness ≤30 min
4. Bony enlargement of knee on examination
5. Age ≥38 yr
Diagnosis requires 1 + 2 + 4, or 1 + 2 + 3 + 5, or 1 + 4 + 5

Knee: Clinical and Radiographic
1. Knee pain for most days of prior month
2. Osteophytes at joint margins
3. Synovial fluid typical of OA
4. Age ≥40 yr
5. Morning stiffness ≤30 min
6. Crepitus with active joint motion
Diagnosis requires 1 + 2, or 1 + 3 + 5 + 6, or 1 + 4 + 5 + 6

Hand
1. Hand pain, aching or stiffness on most days of prior month
2. Hard tissue enlargement of ≥2 of 10 selected joints*
3. Fewer than 3 swollen MCP joints
4. Hard tissue enlargement of ≥2 DIP joints
5. Deformity of ≥2 of 10 selected joints
Diagnosis requires 1–3 and either 4 or 5

Hip: Clinical and Radiographic
1. Hip pain for most days of prior month
2. ESR ≤20 mm/hr
3. Radiographic femoral and/or acetabular osteophytes
4. Radiographic hip joint space narrowing
Diagnosis requires 1 + 2 + 3, or 1 + 2 + 4, or 1 + 3 + 4

***10 selected joints:** 2–3 DIP, 2–3 PIP, CMC bilaterally
CMC: Carpometacarpal; DIP: Distal interphalangeal; ESR: Erythrocyte sedimentation rate; MCP: metacarpophalangeal; PIP: Proximal interphalangeal

Conventional radiographs of the affected joints reveal joint space narrowing, eburnation, subchondral cysts and osteophytes. In early stages, MRI may pick up degenerative changes in bone, cartilage and meniscus and may show mild synovitis.

Treatment

Management of OA includes non-pharmacological, pharmacological and surgeries. Non-pharmacological treatment includes:

a. Patient education regarding the disease, its chronicity and the importance of self-management.
b. Reduction of weight–even a 5% reduction in weight leads to a marked improvement in symptoms.
c. Avoiding excessive loading.
d. Strengthening of surrounding muscles by guided exercises.
e. Braces, splints or canes can be used for unloading the joints in later stages of the disease or when the joint is unstable.

Pharmacological interventions are given in Table 27.2.

Nutraceuticals like glucosamine, chondroitin and immunomodulators are not recommended.

Intra-articular viscosupplementation has been used with variable results in patients awaiting or refusing joint replacement surgeries but is not recommended.

Platelet-rich plasma and mesenchymal stem cell therapies remain unproven.

Surgical interventions for OA include corrective surgeries and joint replacement surgeries.

Some of the upcoming drugs for OA are anti-nerve growth factor (NGF) monoclonal antibody (tanezumab) and drug modulating Wnt signalling pathway (lorecivivint). Other targets for drug development in OA are IL-1 and MMPs (matrix metalloproteinases).

Table 27.2: Pharmacological interventions				
Drug Name	*Route*	*Indications*	*Toxicity/ Contraindications*	*Special Notes*
NSAIDs/ Acetaminophen	Oral/local application	Used for relieving pain as well as combating inflammation	Gastrointestinal ulceration/ perforation Coronary artery disease Stage 3–5 renal disease	To be used cautiously in elders and for short durations
Corticosteroids	Intra-articular	Severe local inflammation of a particular joint	High doses may cause avascular necrosis of the joint	Helpful for controlling flares
Colchicine	Oral	Presence of intra-articular crystals especially calcium pyrophosphate dihydrate	Diarrhea is intolerable in a few	Helpful in controlling inflammation and thus pain
Duloxetine	Oral	Pain hypersensitivity and chronic widespread pain	Constipation, dry mouth, dizziness, insomnia	

Prognosis

OA is a chronic, progressive disease that substantially affects the quality of life. Timely interventions by an integrated team can reduce the progression of disability and blunt the increase in mortality.

Clinical Snippet

A 45-year-old overweight female presenting with gradually increasing knee pain on activity from 3 years. Examination of knee joints revealed crepitus and restricted range of motion with no swelling. A radiograph of both knees revealed reduced joint space in the medial compartment, subchondral sclerosis and osteophytes. The patient was advised to reduce weight, do muscle-strengthening exercises and avoid squatting. She was prescribed NSAIDs for on-demand use and supplemented with calcium and vitamin D.

FURTHER READING

1. GBD 2021 Osteoarthritis Collaborators. Global, regional, and national burden of osteoarthritis, 1990-2020 and projections to 2050: a systematic analysis for the Global Burden of Disease Study 2021. Lancet Rheumatol. 2023 Aug 21;5(9):e508-e522. doi: 10.1016/S2665-9913(23)00163–7.
2. Kolasinski SL, Neogi T, Hochberg, et al. 2019 American College of Rheumatology/Arthritis Foundation Guideline for the Management of Osteoarthritis of the Hand, Hip, and Knee. Arthritis Care Res (Hoboken). 2020 Feb;72(2):149-162. doi: 10.1002/acr.24131.

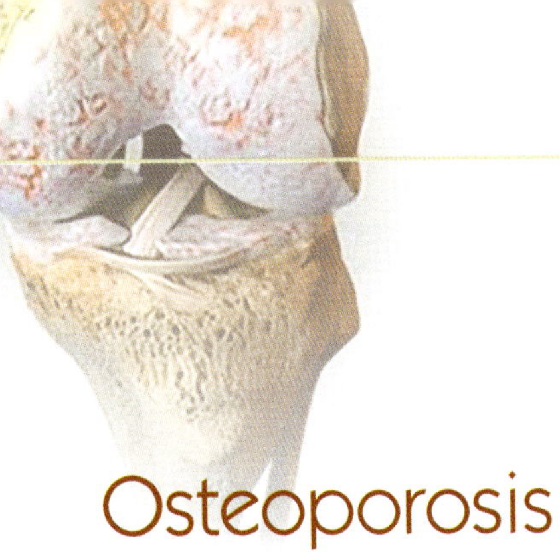

Osteoporosis

Parthajit Das

INTRODUCTION

Osteoporosis is a skeletal disease characterised by reduced bone strength due to low bone mineral density (BMD) and bone microarchitecture, leading to an augmented risk of fracture. It is assumed that more than 25 million people are having osteoporosis in India.

Aetiology

Primary osteoporosis is associated with age and sex hormone deficiency as found in postmenopausal women and ageing men. Secondary osteoporosis is associated with several medical conditions and/or medications (Table 28.1).

Clinical Features and Risk Factors

Osteoporosis is a silent disease in the early phases. However, a wide range of clinical presentations may be attributed to osteoporosis such as back pain caused by vertebral fractures (VF), height loss over time, stooped posture, nontraumatic nonvertebral fractures, etc.

Diagnosis

The gold standard for diagnosis incorporates BMD measurements in the lumbar spine, hip and distal radius with the dual-energy X-ray absorptiometry or the occurrence of

Table 28.1: Causes of secondary osteoporosis in adults	
Endocrine	Acromegaly, diabetes mellitus, hypogonadism, hyperparathyroidism, hyperthyroidism,
Gastrointestinal	Alcoholism, anorexia nervosa, malabsorption syndrome, IBD
Drugs	Antiepileptics, aromatase inhibitors, glucocorticoids, heparin, chemotherapeutic agents, SGLT2 inhibitors, lithium
Collagen metabolism	Ehlers-Danlos syndrome, osteogenesis imperfecta
Respiratory	COPD
Rheumatology	Rheumatoid arthritis, SLE, ankylosing spondylitis, polymyositis
Renal	Renal insufficiency, renal tubular acidosis, transplantation
Hematology	Thalassemia, hemophilia, multiple myeloma
Others	AIDS/HIV, major depression

Table 28.2: T-Scores and WHO diagnostic criteria for osteoporosis	
Interpretation	T-score
Normal	–1.0 and higher
Osteopenia	–1.0 to –2.5
Osteoporosis	–2.5 and lower
Severe osteoporosis	–2.5 and lower with one or more fragility fractures

nontraumatic hip or vertebral fractures (Table 28.2). Although it is convenient to estimate BMD, optimum assessment of bone quality remains a challenge. T-scores compare BMD with that of a healthy person, whereas Z-scores use the average BMD of people of the same age, sex, and size as a comparator. Vertebral fracture assessment, a component of DXA imaging, is considered a better prediction tool for the detection of VF. Trabecular bone score is an indirect measure of microarchitecture and could be obtained from DXA images of the lumbar spine.

The best-suited modalities of measuring volumetric BMD include high-resolution micro-computed tomography (micro CT) and micro-magnetic resonance imaging (micro MRI) that illustrates the 3D characterization of bone microarchitecture along with BMD and estimation of fracture risk.

Bone turnover markers have a limited role in the diagnosis. Bone formation markers (Procollagen type I N-terminal propeptide-P1NP) or resorption markers (C telopeptide of Type 1 collagen-CTx) with DXA can be used to identify high-risk patients for future fracture, monitor treatment compliance and response, or plan for drug holidays.

The National Osteoporosis Foundation recommends monitoring BMD one to two years after initiation of treatment and every two years thereafter.

Fracture Risk Assessment

The absolute risk of fracture can be calculated using a prediction tool, such as FRAX (fracture risk assessment tool) (www.shef.ac.uk/frax/). By combining several risk factors for osteoporosis with DXA results, the 10-year risk of major osteoporotic fracture and hip fracture for patients more than 40 years of age is estimated. FRAXplus® gives a more accurate risk assessment by including more factors.

Treatment of Osteoporosis

Treatment recommendations vary widely. Clinical use, efficacy data and toxicities of FDA-approved osteoporosis medicines are discussed in Table 28.3.

- Lifestyle recommendations include smoking cessation, moderation of alcohol intake, habitual weight-bearing exercises or resistance training, and assessment and prevention of fall risk.
- Recommended dietary and supplemented elemental calcium intake is up to 1000 to 1200 mg daily in adults (1000–1300 mg daily in children), whereas vitamin D intake is 600–800 IU/day.
- Anabolic or antiresorptive agents are both commonly used in clinical practice. Sequential therapy with an antiresorptive agent following treatment with an anabolic agent is strongly recommended to mitigate rapid bone loss and enhanced VF rate. Raloxifene (a selective oestrogen-receptor modulator- SERM) and calcitonin should be reserved for patients in whom other treatments have failed or are contraindicated.

Table 28.3: FDA approved medicines in osteoporosis

Compound	Dosing/Strength	Route-Frequency	Side effects	2-yr increase in spine BMD	2-yr increase in total Hip BMD
Antiresorptive Agents					
Bisphosphonates (BPs)		Oral—daily/weekly	Heart burn, stomach pain, osteonecrosis of jaw(ONG)-rare, atypical femoral fracture (AFF)—rare	Oral BPs 3–5%	Oral BPs 2–3%
Alendronate	10 mg/70 mg	Oral—weekly			
Risedronate	35 mg	Oral/Intravenous—monthly, every 3 months			
Ibandronate	150 mg/1 mg per ml—3mg vial	Oral/Intravenous—monthly, every 3 months			
Zoledronate	5 mg palpitations	Intravenous—every 12 months	allergic reactions, arthralgia, myalgia, infection, ONJ (rare)	5–6%	3–4%
RANKL inhibitor					
Denosumab	60 mg	Subcutaneous—every 6 months	Arthralgia, allergic reaction, hypocalcemia, infections, ONJ (rare), AFF (rare)	6–8%	3–4%
Estrogen agonist/Antagonist					
Raloxifene	60 mg	Oral—daily	Hot flashes, leg cramps, venous thromboembolism, and stroke	2–3%	1%
Conjugated estrogens/ bazedoxifene	0.45 mg/20 mg	Oral—daily			
ANABOLIC AGENTS					
Parathyroid Hormone Analogues					
Teriparatide	20 µg	Subcutaneous—daily	Constipation, arthralgia, chest pain, hypercalcemia, possible malignancy risk in animal models	8–10%	1.5–2%
Abaloparatide	80 µg	Subcutaneous—daily	Orthostatic hypotension, hypercalcemia, urolithiasis.	10%	2–3%
Sclerostin inhibitors					
Romosozumab	210 mg	Subcutaneous—monthly	(MI, Cardiovascular death), AFF (rare), ONJ (rare), hypocalcemia	11% (1yr)	4% (1 yr)

- Several newer osteoporosis agents such as abaloparatide (a synthetic peptide analogue of the human parathyroid hormone-related peptide), romosozumab (a humanized monoclonal antibody to sclerostin), bazedoxifene (a third-generation SERM), balicatib and ONO-5334 (Cathepsin K inhibitor) have demonstrated promising results.

Treatment Failure

Treatment failure should be considered if there are 2 or more incident fragility fractures, 1 incident fracture *plus* significant (>Least Significant Change) decrease BMD *or* inadequate suppression BTM, no fracture but *both* a decrease in BMD *and* inadequate suppression BTM.

Osteoporosis in Special Populations

- Pregnancy-related osteoporosis is characterized by the occurrence of fracture during pregnancy or the puerperium. Although there are concerns about fetal toxicity therapeutic agents with shorter half-life such as risedronate and teriparatide are generally recommended.
- In children, osteoporosis is uncommon and is defined by the presence of both history of pathologic fractures and low BMD. The occurrence of a single significant fracture in a long bone of the lower extremity, two fractures in the long bone of an upper extremity, or one vertebral compression fracture fulfils the diagnostic criterion. Z scores of –2 standard deviation define low bone mass for age.
- Glucocorticoid-induced osteoporosis—prolonged glucocorticoid use harms the bone mass. Fracture risk is increased even at daily doses of prednisolone/equivalent as low as 2.5 to 7.5 mg. As per ACR guidelines, If glucocorticoid dose is > 7.5 mg/day, multiply the 10-year risk of major osteoporotic fracture by 1.15 and the hip fracture risk by 1.2
- Renal transplant with CKD-When eGFR <35 ml/min, CKD MBD should be excluded. Once excluded, no dose adjustment is required while prescribing denosumab, teriparatide/abaloparatide, or romosozumab, but avoid bisphosphonates.

Conclusion

Osteoporosis is a worldwide concern. Early diagnosis with advanced technologies, lifestyle modifications, appropriate risk stratification and judicious use of contemporary and novel osteoporosis agents in sequence or combination could minimize morbidity, mortality and burdens of living with osteoporosis.

FURTHER READING

1. Gregson CL, Armstrong DJ, Bowden J, Cooper C, Edwards J, Gittoes NJL, Harvey N, Kanis J, Leyland S, Low R, McCloskey E, Moss K, Parker J, Paskins Z, Poole K, Reid DM, Stone M, Thomson J, Vine N, Compston J. UK clinical guideline for the prevention and treatment of osteoporosis. Arch Osteoporos. 2022 Apr 5;17(1):58.
2. Humphrey MB, Russell L, Danila MI, Fink HA, Guyatt G, Cannon M, Caplan L, Gore S, Grossman J, Hansen KE, Lane NE, Ma NS, Magrey M, McAlindon T, Robinson AB, Saha S, Womack C, Abdulhadi B, Charles JF, Cheah JTL, Chou S, Goyal I, Haseltine K, Jackson L, Mirza R, Moledina I, Punni E, Rinden T, Turgunbaev M, Wysham K, Turner AS, Uhl S. 2022 American College of Rheumatology Guideline for the Prevention and Treatment of Glucocorticoid-Induced Osteoporosis. Arthritis Rheumatol. 2023 Dec;75(12):2088–2102.

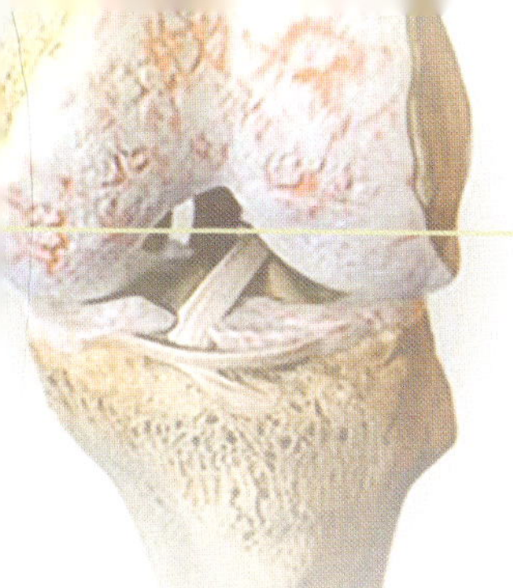

Paget's Disease of Bone

Emil J Thachil

INTRODUCTION

Paget's disease of bone (PDB) is a metabolic bone disease, next only to osteoporosis. Defective remodelling process leading to abnormal soft, deformed enlarged bones characterize the disease. First described as osteitis deformans by Sir James Paget (1876), it is more common after 40 years and seen more in males.

Exact cause is unknown. Mutations in gene encoding the scaffolding protein p62 Sequestosome 1 *(SQSTM1)* with a role in nuclear factor kappa-B (NF-kB) pathway has been linked to familial Paget's. A viral cause (especially paramyxovirus) affecting osteoclast function has been suggested as demonstrated by inclusion bodies in the Paget's osteoclasts, but no virus has been isolated yet.

There are aberrant overactive large osteoclasts causing focal and excessive bone resorption. Compensatory bone formation by osteoblasts is disorganised leading to deformed abnormally large but soft bone. This process occurs in three characteristic phases: Osteolytic, mixed lytic-sclerotic and osteosclerotic.

Clinical Features

Bone involvement is usually focal with polyostotic distribution being more common. There is an axial predilection with the pelvis being the most common site. Other sites include spine (especially lumbar), femur, tibia, skull and hip in descending order of involvement. PDB is typically diagnosed after an evaluation for an abnormal radiograph, or an abnormally high alkaline phosphatase (ALP) found during evaluation for other reasons. Patients most often present with musculoskeletal complaints including localised bone pains, deformities (protrusio acetabuli, bowing, frontal bossing), pathological fractures, osteoarthritis, etc. Less than 1% may develop secondary osteosarcoma.

Neurological manifestations due to compression such as headaches, obstructive hydrocephalus and cranial neuropathies causing deafness, visual loss, etc. have been described. Presentations due to increased metabolic turnover such as high output cardiac failure and gout may also be encountered.

Diagnosis

The easiest available marker for disease activity assessment and therapeutic monitoring is serum alkaline phosphatase which if raised initially can be used for regular monitoring. It may remain normal in monostotic and early polyostotic disease. Calcium, phosphorus, parathyroid hormone and vitamin D all may remain normal. Among bone turnover markers, the best marker for activity assessment and monitoring disease is serum procollagen type 1 N-terminal propeptide (P1NP). Other useful alternatives include bone specific ALP and urine N-terminal telopeptide.

Imaging

Conventional radiograph is enough in most cases for diagnosis and will show a mixture of focal lytic lesions with sclerosis (mosaic bone pattern) and in later stages bone enlargement. Lesion will not spread beyond the involved bone. Pseudofractures have been described. Fractures are typically transverse due to weak bone architecture, referred to as 'chalk stick fractures or banana fractures.' Radiological imaging findings are tabulated (*see* Table 29.1). Bone scan can help to confirm polyostotic disease and localize the involved sites.

Treatment

Early treatment for PDB is required in symptomatic patients and those at risk of complications or deformities as they are irreversible. All patients should receive calcium and vitamin D supplementation daily.

Preferred first line agents for PDB are bisphosphonates. The available options are tabulated (*see* Table 29.2). Zoledronic acid may be considered the drug of choice

Table 29.1: Radiological findings in Paget's disease

Site	Radiological sign	Description
Skull	Osteoporosis circumscripta	Circumscribed lytic lesions.
	Moth eaten appearance	Multiple endosteal lucencies
	Tam o' Shanter sign	Cranial bones over-riding the facial bones similar to Tam o' Shanter hat.
	Cotton wool appearance	Lucent areas of the calvarium containing fluffy sclerotic trabecula.
Pelvis	Brim sign	Sclerosis along the iliopectineal and ischiopubic lines
Spine	Picture frame vertebrae	Thickened vertebral body cortex.
	Ivory vertebrae	Normal sized body but diffuse, homogeneously increased opacity.
Long bones	Blade of grass appearance (Candle flame sign)	Wedge-shaped areas of resorption.

Table 29.2: Bisphosphonates in treatment of Paget's disease of bone

Bisphosphonates	Dosage	Duration	MOA	Biochemical remission (normalisation of ALP at 6 months)	Adverse effects
Zoledronic acid	5 mg	Single dose	IV	89%	GI: Diarrhea, abdominal pain Hypocalcemia Fever, myalgia with IV infusions Increased risk for subtrochanteric fractures and osteonecrosis of jaw
Risedronate	30 mg/day	2 months	Oral	58%	
Alendronate	40 mg/day	6 months	Oral	48%	
Pamidronate	60 mg/day	3 days	IV		

considering the fast and sustained therapeutic response. Relapses were more with Risedronate as against zoledronate (20% vs 0.7%). Retreatment may be needed if markers remain high. Bisphosphonates are contraindicated in renal impairment.

Teriparatide trials showed increased risk for osteosarcoma in rats and may not be advisable in PDB. Calcitonin is useful only to relieve bone pains. Denosumab has been reported to be effective in few case reports. It can be considered as a second-line option in those where bisphosphonates are contraindicated only if long term efficacy and safety can be properly established. Deformities may need corrective surgeries.

Prognosis

Overall prognosis is good in early stages and monostotic PDB. Five year survival of PDB with osteosarcomatous change is very poor (<8%).

FURTHER READING

1. Banaganapalli B, Fallatah I, Alsubhi F, Shetty PJ, Awan Z, Elango R and Shaik NA (2023) Paget's disease: a review of the epidemiology, etiology, genetics, and treatment. *Front. Genet.* 14:1131182. doi: 10.3389/fgene.2023.1131182.
2. Smith S, Murphey M, Motamedi K, Mulligan M, Resnik C, Gannon F. From the Archives of the AFIP. Radiologic Spectrum of Paget Disease of Bone and Its Complications with Pathologic Correlation. Radiographics. 2002;22(5):1191–216.
3. Reid, I. Management of Paget's disease of bone. *Osteoporos Int* 31, 827–837 (2020). https://doi.org/10.1007/s00198-019-05259-1.

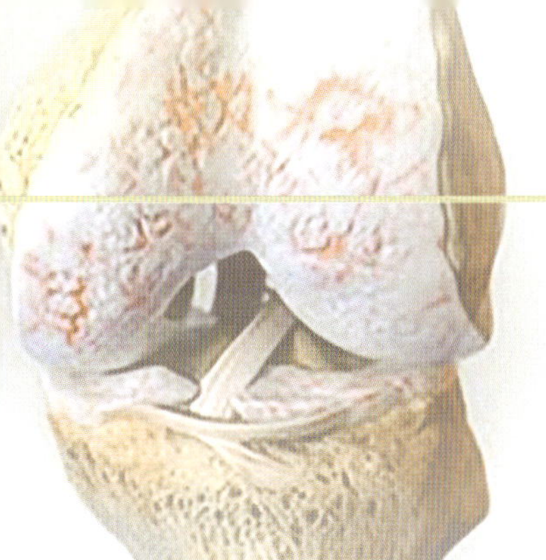

Other Connective Tissue Diseases and Manifestations

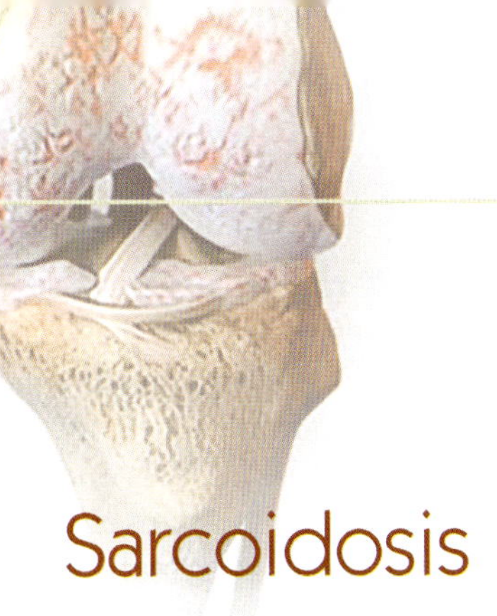

Sarcoidosis

Arun Kumar Kedia

INTRODUCTION

Sarcoidosis is a multisystem disorder of unknown etiology characterized by noncaseating granulomas in various organs. Associations with occupational and environmental exposures to beryllium, dust, and different microorganisms like mycobacteria and propionibacteria have been described.

Genetic susceptibility is usually related to the major histocompatibility complex (MHC) antigens, especially DR alleles. Cytokines, including interleukins, interferon (IFN) gamma, and tumor necrosis factor (TNF) alpha are implicated in granuloma formation with macrophage and epithelioid accumulation, activation, and aggregation. Additionally, B cell hyperreactivity with immunoglobulin production is also implicated.

The exact incidence in India is unknown. While 90% of cases have pulmonary involvement, extrapulmonary sarcoid is seen in up to 25 to 30% of patients with cardiac involvement which is more common in males, while skin and eye features are more prominent in women.

Clinical Features

Symptoms are variable and depend on the organ involvement. Though it typically presents with bilateral hilar lymphadenopathy and reticular opacities in the lungs, it can manifest to a variable degree in the musculoskeletal system, reticuloendothelial system, exocrine glands, heart, kidney, and central nervous system.

Pulmonary involvement in 90% of cases is detected incidentally on routine chest radiography before patients present clinically, with a persistent dry cough, fatigue, chest pain, and shortness of breath. Upper airway involvement may be seen with submucosal granuloma in the larynx, pharynx, and sinuses. Endobronchial and lower airway involvement can lead to airway narrowing and chronic cases can progress to lung fibrosis and pulmonary hypertension.

Rheumatological manifestations include arthropathy, myopathy, bone lesions, and vasculitis in rare cases. Acute sarcoid arthritis is mainly oligoarticular, occasionally polyarticular, and rarely monoarticular. It commonly involves ankles and knees and may be mistaken for reactive arthritis. Other joints may be involved similar to RA. It usually carries a good prognosis with spontaneous resolution within 3–6 months. Lofgren's syndrome is characterized by the triad of hilar adenopathy on chest X-ray, acute arthritis (usually bilateral ankles), and erythema nodosum. Only 15% of cases especially those with raised ACE levels may have persistent arthritis. Chronic arthritis is rare and may present as non-deforming arthritis with granulomatous synovitis or a non-erosive joint deformity. These cases may have parenchymal lung disease with raised ACE levels and are often positive for rheumatoid factor. Dactylitis involving 2nd and 3rd phalanges and tenosynovitis may also occur. Myopathies, though rare may be a presenting feature. Patients may present with insidious onset of symmetrical proximal muscle weakness with normal or raised muscle enzymes, acute myopathy, or nodular painful myopathy. Acute myopathy may involve the diaphragm and lead to acute respiratory failure. Bone involvement is usually asymptomatic and can vary from cystic, lytic, and sclerotic to focal bone lesions. They are usually detected on routine X-rays or sometimes on MRI. The presence of bone involvement is suggestive of chronic severe sarcoidosis with chronic lung and multiorgan involvement. Vasculitis is rare and can involve small, medium, and large arteries and may be a life-threatening presenting feature.

Amongst the most common cutaneous lesions are papular sarcoidosis involving the upper half of the face, the back of the neck, and previous trauma, scar sites, and tattoos. Lupus pernio is a variant that presents with violaceous or erythematous papules, plaques, or nodules, mainly involving the central facial skin. Erythema nodosum presents with painful nodules (due to panniculitis) on shins and is a part of Löfgren syndrome.

Ocular manifestations are seen in nearly 50% of patients, of which the most common clinical feature is uveitis. Other manifestations include keratoconjunctivitis which in association with salivary gland involvement may mimic Sjögrens syndrome. Heerfordt's syndrome is a combination of anterior uveitis, parotid enlargement, facial palsy and fever.

Hypercalciuria and hypercalcemia leading to nephrocalcinosis and renal failure may be seen with unregulated hypersecretion of Vit D from granulomas. Some patients may present with peripheral lymphadenopathy and hepatosplenomegaly due to granulomas in reticuloendothelial organs.

Heart block, ventricular arrhythmias, and sudden death due to cardiac involvement have also been reported and prophylactic insertion of an implantable cardioverter-defibrillator (ICD) is recommended in such patients. CNS manifestations include Psychiatric manifestations, seizures, diabetes insipidus, hyperprolactinemia, lymphocytic meningitis, and cranial nerve palsies.

Diagnosis

There is no diagnostic test specific for sarcoidosis. Initial evaluation includes CBP and differential looking for anemia of chronic disease, lymphopenia, thrombocytopenia, liver function tests, blood urea nitrogen, creatinine, glucose, electrolytes, and serum calcium looking for hypercalcemia. ESR and CRP are nonspecific but may be elevated. Elevated serum ALP concentration suggests diffuse granulomatous hepatic involvement. Serum angiotensin-converting enzyme (ACE) may be elevated in chronic cases. Imaging tests include chest X-ray PA view and CT of the chest. Cardiac or CNS-affected sarcoidosis is better diagnosed with the help of an MRI or PET scan. Pulmonary function tests and echocardiography may aid in diagnosing the progression of lung disease.

A biopsy is often required to confirm the diagnosis. Transbronchial biopsy has a high yield. If that fails, then a mediastinoscopy to perform a lymph node biopsy is required. The key feature is noncaseating granulomas in the absence of mycobacteria and fungi.

Treatment

Sarcoidosis has no obvious cause, and hence prevention is not possible. The disorder also resolves spontaneously in 30–70% of cases; hence, treatment is not always required.

Steroids are the cornerstone of the therapy and symptomatic patients need good compliance and follow-up to monitor adverse side effects. Patients who fail to respond to steroids may need potent biological agents and DMARDs. Methotrexate, antimalarials, cyclophosphamide, azathioprine and cyclosporine can be used as second-line therapy or as steroid-sparing agents.

Prognosis

Overall, about one-fifth of patients develop progressive functional impairment, and there is a mortality rate of 3 to 5% in patients who are not adequately treated. Adverse effects of long-term steroid therapy also need consideration during follow-up.

FURTHER READING

1. Sève P, Pacheco Y, Durupt F, Jamilloux Y, Gerfaud-Valentin M, Isaac S, et al. Sarcoidosis: A Clinical Overview from Symptoms to Diagnosis. Cells. 2021 Mar 31;10(4):766.
2. Llanos O, Hamzeh N. Sarcoidosis. Med Clin North Am. 2019 May;103(3):527–534.
3. Kobak S. Sarcoidosis: a rheumatologist's perspective. Ther Adv Musculoskelet Dis. 2015 Oct;7(5):196–205.

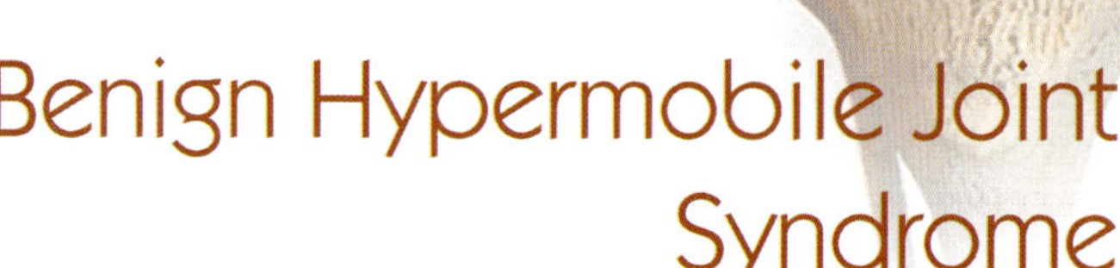

Benign Hypermobile Joint Syndrome

Kshiti Rai, NV Jayachandran

INTRODUCTION

Benign hypermobile joint syndrome (BHJS) is a connective tissue disorder with hypermobility in which musculoskeletal symptoms occur in the absence of systemic rheumatologic disease. It is characterised by generalised ligamentous laxity and the presence of musculoskeletal pain. BHJS is a relatively common phenomenon with a prevalence ranging from 5 to 18% in Caucasian populations and up to 43% in non-Caucasian populations. Hypermobility may occur in several different connective tissue disorders including Marfan syndrome, Ehlers-Danlos syndrome and osteogenesis imperfecta. It may also be found in chromosomal and genetic disorders such as Down syndrome and in metabolic disorders such as homocystinuria and hyperlysinemia.

Clinical Features

The signs and symptoms of BHJS are variable. Most commonly, the initial complaint in a hypermobile patient is joint pain, which may affect one or multiple joints and may be generalised or symmetric, usually precipitated by physical activity. The joint pains are a result of unrecognised micro-trauma. Besides joint pains, patients present with enthesitis, bursitis, tenosynovitis, chondromalacia patellae, rotator cuff problems and mechanical back pain. Patients are at increased risk of recurrent joint dislocations, subluxations and sprains as a result of joint instability. Some patients may develop correctable deformities of joints without ever suffering from arthritis. Findings of the physical examination vary based on the joints affected. Pain in response to manipulation of the joint is common. The presence of clinically significant joint tenderness, redness, swelling, or warmth indicating signs of inflammation are absent in patients with BHJS. Several studies have noted the association of joint hypermobility with primary fibromyalgia. Besides bones and joints, these patients may have other extra-articular manifestations such as mitral valve prolapse, hernias and prolapse of rectum and uterus, psychiatric manifestations like depression, anxiety and panic attacks. Reduced vascular stiffness predisposes to risk of varicose veins, and eye involvement may contribute to high myopia.

Diagnosis

For initial assessment of joint hypermobility, Beighton score (Table 31.1) has to be determined. A Beighton score of 4 or more points is indicative of generalised joint laxity.

To establish the diagnosis of BHJS, Brighton criteria (Box 31.1) is used which also helps in distinguishing it from other connective tissue disorders. Evaluation should be directed at exclusion of other heritable disorders of connective tissues that are associated with hypermobility.

Treatment

The management of patients with BHJS can be challenging for the patient as well as the practitioner. As described by Simmonds and Keer, "patience, coupled with good communication and sensitive handling skills are required as physical problems are often long-standing and include secondary complications and psycho-social issues." There is no conclusive evidence in the literature regarding best practices for patients with BHJS. However, patient education, therapeutic exercise, modification of work and lifestyle, joint protection, and proper body mechanics in the management of BHJS is of

Table 31.1: Beighton score		
Description	*Bilateral Testing*	*Scoring (maximum points)*
1. Passive dorsiflexion and hyperextension of the fifth MCP joint beyond 90°	Yes	2
2. Passive apposition of the thumb to the flexor aspect of the forearm	Yes	2
3. Passive hyperextension of the elbow beyond 10°	Yes	2
4. Passive hyperextension of the knee beyond 10°	Yes	2
5. Active forward flexion of the trunk with the knees fully extended so that the palms of the hands rest flat on the floor	No	1
Total		9

Box 31.1: Brighton criteria

Major criteria

1. A Beighton score of 4/9 or greater (currently or historically)
2. Arthralgia for 3 months in 4 or more joints

Minor criteria

1. A Beighton score of 1, 2 or 3/9 (0, 1, 2, or 3 if aged 50+)
2. Arthralgia (≥3 months) in 1–3 joints, or back pain ≥3 months, spondylosis, spondylolysis/spondylolisthesis
3. Dislocation/subluxation in one or more joints or in one joint on more than one occasion
4. Soft tissue rheumatism ≥3 lesions (e.g., epicondylitis, tenosynovitis, bursitis)
5. Marfanoid habitus (tall, slim, span/height ratio >1.03, upper:lower segment ratio <0.89, arachnodactyly [+Steinberg/wrist signs])
6. Abnormal skin: Striae, hyperextensibility, thin skin, papyraceous, or scarring
7. Eye signs: Drooping eyelids or myopia or antimongoloid slant
8. Varicose veins, hernia/rectal prolapse

utmost importance. The objective of the exercise therapy is to strengthen and stabilise the hypermobile joints and thereby protect the joints from microtrauma. Exercise therapy should be under the supervision of experienced physiotherapists.

Prognosis

The prognosis for patients with BJHS is generally good owing to the syndrome's nonprogressive nature and decreased joint laxity that occur with age. However, patients need to be aware of the potential sequelae and associations. This underscores the importance of making an early diagnosis and educating the patient.

Clinical Snippet

A 28-year-old female from Kozhikode, Kerala, presented with pain in bilateral knee joints and shoulder joints for the past 6 months, due to which her daily activities were disturbed. However, the pain did not have any diurnal variation, no associated redness and swelling of the joint, no stiffness in joint after prolonged sitting. There was no significant family history of joint hypermobility or a significant medical history in the past.

On clinical examination, height-147 cm, weight-45 kg (BMI-20.83), arm span-149 cm (arm span > height), upper segment-79 cm, and lower segment-70 cm (upper segment: lower segment ratio-1.12). Skin and hair were normal. Systemic examination and lab parameters were within normal limits. Her Beighton score was 6/9. Based on history, clinical examination, and laboratory tests, she was diagnosed as having BHJS. She was treated with therapeutic exercise and proper joint mechanics and is doing well till date.

FURTHER READING

1. Simpson MMR. Benign Joint Hypermobility Syndrome: Evaluation, Diagnosis, and Management. J Am Osteopath Assoc. 2006;106(9):531–36.
2. Grahame R. The revised (Brighton 1998) criteria for the diagnosis of benign joint hypermobility syndrome (BJHS). J Rheumatol. 2000;27:1777–1779.
3. Russek LN. Examination and treatment of a patient with hypermobility syndrome. *Phys Ther.* 2000;80:386–98.

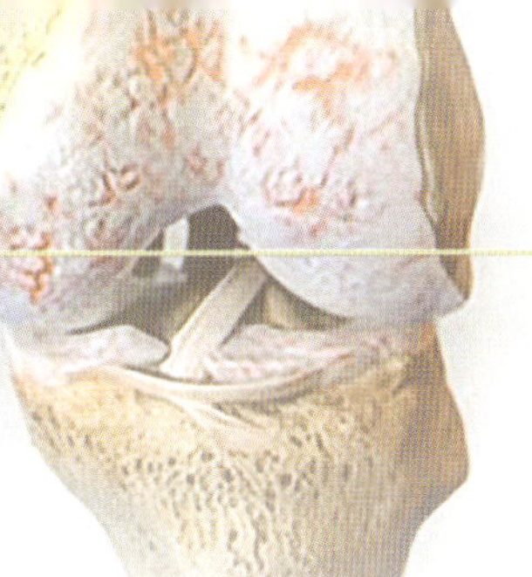

IgG4 Related Disease: An Overview

Amit Dua, Lalit Duggal

INTRODUCTION

IgG4-related disease (IgG4-RD) is a systemic fibroinflammatory condition characterized by tumefactive lesions, increased serum IgG4 levels, and distinctive histopathological features. This review aims to provide an in-depth evaluation of IgG4-RD.

The disease has been reported worldwide, with a higher prevalence in Asia (particularly Japan and South Korea). Global prevalence of IGG4 RD is 0.28–1.08 per 100,000 people and Prevalence in Asia is 0.42–1.46 per 100,000 people. The incidence of IgG4 RD worldwide is 0.02–0.11 per 100,000 person-years whereas its incidence in Asia is 0.04–0.14 per 100,000 person-years. It is mostly seen in middle to old age patients with a peak incidence between 50 to 70 years of age (male: female ratio, 1.3–1.5: 1).

The pathogenesis of IgG4-RD involves a complex interplay of immune cells, cytokines, and fibroblasts. IgG4 antibodies play a central role in the disease, although their exact mechanism of action remains unclear. Genetic susceptibility and environmental triggers lead to immune system activation that provokes the pathogenesis of the disease. These factors are discussed in Fig. 32.1.

Genetic Predisposition

1. HLA-DRB1 polymorphisms
2. CTLA-4 polymorphisms
3. Familial cases indicate potential genetic component

Environmental Triggers

1. Infections
2. Autoantigens (e.g., pancreatic antigens)
3. Other environmental factors (e.g., smoking)

Immune System Activation

Antigens (e.g., infections, autoantigens) are presented to T-cells by antigen-presenting cells (APCs). APCs (dendritic cells, macrophages) process and present antigens via MHC molecules. Activation of CD4+ T-cells and Th2 cytokine profile, promotes IgG4 production and fibrosis. Activated T-cells also interact with B-cells

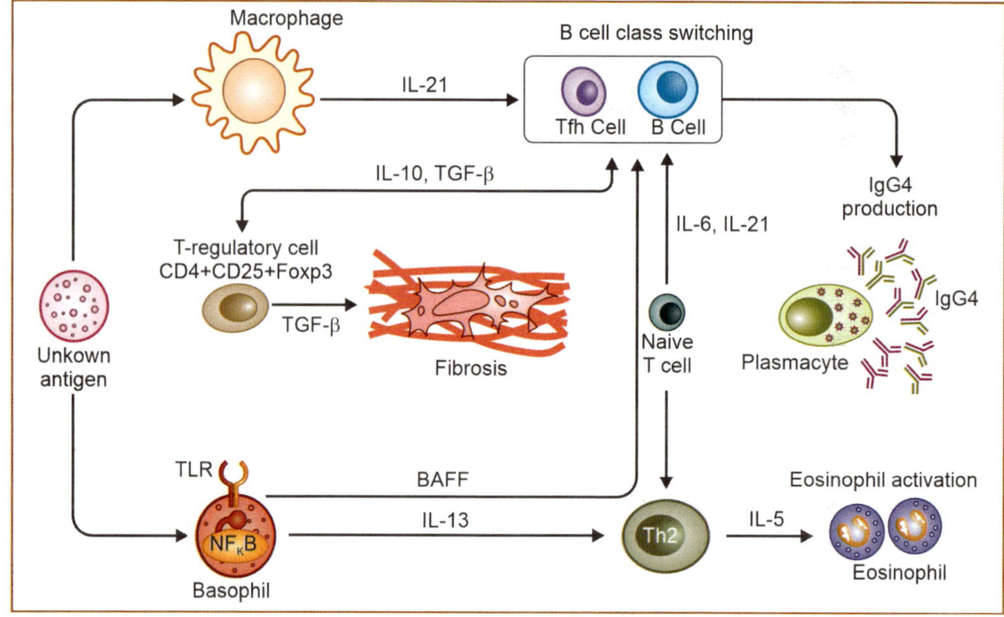

Fig 32.1: Schematic pathogenesis model of IgG4-related disease

and activate them. B-cells recognize antigens and undergo class-switching to IgG4. It also leads to ectopic germinal center formation which produce autoantibodies and causes tissue destruction.

Clinical Features

IgG4-RD can affect nearly every structure of the body but mostly involves lacrimal and salivary glands, thyroid gland, pancreas, bile ducts, retroperitoneum, kidney aorta, meninges, and lymph nodes. Multiple organs are involved in 60 to 90% of patients. The disease commonly has a subacute presentation. It can present as mass forming lesions which can lead to permanent organ damage and can be fatal if left untreated. This is a great mimicker of many malignant, infectious and inflammatory conditions. Fever (50–60%), fatigue (40–50%), and weight loss (30–40%) are the common systemic symptoms of IgG RD patients. Clinical features of IgG4-RD also vary depending on the affected organ (Tables 32.1 and 32.2).

Diagnosis of IgG4-RD requires a combination of:
1. Clinical features as described in Tables 32.3 and 32.4
2. Serological feature—elevated serum IgG4 levels (>135 mg/dL)
3. Imaging studies (CT, MRI, USG and PET)
4. Histopathological examination/biopsy

Pathological Features of IgG4-RD

1. Dense lymphoplasmacytic inflammation-IgG4-positive plasma cell infiltration
2. Fibrosis with a storiform pattern
3. Obstructive phlebitis
   Granulomas are uncommon, and the presentation makes the diagnosis unlikely.

Table 32.1: Organ involvement and clinical features of IgG4-RD

Organ	Clinical features	Frequency
Pancreas	Abdominal pain, jaundice, weight loss, pancreatic enlargement	60–70%
Salivary glands	Swelling, pain, xerostomia, parotid gland enlargement	50–60%
Biliary tract	Jaundice, abdominal pain, cholangitis, bile duct narrowing	30–40%
Kidneys	Nephrotic syndrome, renal failure, kidney enlargement	20–30%
Skin	Erythema, nodules, ulcers, skin thickening	10–20%
Eyes	Dacryoadenitis, orbital inflammation, eyelid swelling	10–20%
Lungs	Cough, dyspnea, interstitial lung disease	5–10%
Lymph nodes	Swollen lymph nodes, lymphadenopathy	70–80%
Aorta	Aortitis, aortic aneurysm	5–10%
Breast	Breast swelling, mastitis	5%
Central nervous system	Meningitis, encephalitis, cranial neuropathy	5%

Table 32.2: Imaging findings strongly suggestive of IgG4-RD

Organ	Finding
Pancreas	Pancreatic enlargement/ swelling
Biliary tree	Bile duct narrowing/ stenosis/ strictures
Salivary glands	Enlargement/ swelling
Renal	Enlargement/ swelling
Pulmonary	Infiltrates/ nodules, ILD features

Table 32.3: 2020 Revised comprehensive diagnostic (RCD) criteria for IgG4-RD

Diagnosis	Features	
Possible	Clinical and radiological and serological features	No histopathological confirmation
Probable	Clinical, radiological and pathological features	Not fulfilling the serological criteria
Definite	Clinical, radiological, serological and pathological features	

Table 32.4: Differential diagnosis of IgG4-RD

Category	Conditions
Autoimmune disorders	Sarcoidosis, Sjögren's syndrome, primary sclerosing cholangitis, autoimmune pancreatitis, rheumatoid arthritis, lupus erythematosus, hashimoto's thyroiditis
Inflammatory conditions	Chronic pancreatitis, biliary obstruction, cholangitis, pyelonephritis, interstitial lung disease
Neoplastic conditions	Lymphoma, cancer (pancreatic, biliary, lung), sarcoma
Infectious diseases	Tuberculosis, syphilis, Lyme disease, Cat-scratch disease
Other conditions	Castleman disease, fibromatoses, sclerosing mesenteritis, inflammatory bowel disease

Treatment

Treatment should be individualized based on disease severity, organ involvement, and patient comorbidities.

1. Glucocorticoids are the first-line treatment for IgG4-RD.
2. Immunomodulators and biologic agents may be used as maintenance therapy or for refractory cases.
3. Duration of therapy is not exactly described but it is a common practice to stop maintenance therapy after 2–3 years if in remission.
4. Debulking surgery for obstructive lesions like in ureters, bile ducts, etc.
5. Surgery and radiation therapy may also be considered for refractory cases or complications.
6. Regular monitoring of disease activity, organ function, and treatment side effects is essential.

Prognosis

Nearly all patients respond to steroids but 40% fail to achieve complete remission or can relapse within a year. Higher IgG4 levels, multiorgan involvement, head and neck involvement and stopping steroids are some of the factors responsible for relapse of the disease.

Clinical Snippet

A 34-year-old female came with fever, nausea, vomiting and abdominal pain for 2 months along with sicca symptoms for 1 year. She also had swelling around her left eye and below jaws suggestive of lacrimal and submandibular involvement. She had transaminitis (AST 408 U/L and ALT-450 U/L). Her alkaline phosphatase was 800 U/L. She had increased levels of lipase and amylase. Her viral serology was negative. Other work up for infections was also negative. Her CT abdomen demonstrated a dilated common bile duct, and MRCP confirmed presence of focal stricture of common bile duct near pancreatic head with mesenteric lymphadenopathy. Biopsy was also done during the MRCP, which confirmed a storiform fibrosis and lymphocytic infiltrate. Her ANA, anti-Ro and La were negative. Serum IgG4 levels were 423 mg/dL.

She was diagnosed with IgG4 RD, and treated with prednisolone 30 mg daily. Two doses of rituximab 1 g each were administered 15 days apart. Steroids were tapered over 3 months to 5 mg/day. She responded to the treatment and after 3 months her CT abdomen and pelvis showed resolution of biliary dilatation.

Conclusion

IgG4-related disease (IgG4-RD) is a chronic immune-mediated fibro-inflammatory condition which can present with sclerotic or tumefactive lesions and can affect multiple organs. It can lead to permanent organ damage and can be fatal if left untreated. It is a great-mimicker of many conditions. Histopathologically, it is characterized by lymphoplasmacytic infiltrate rich in IgG4 plasma cells with simultaneous development of storiform fibrosis and obliterative phlebitis. Serum IgG4 levels are often, but not always elevated. Glucocorticoids are the mainstay of treatment. Many steroid sparing conventional agents or biological agent (rituximab) have shown good results. Prompt diagnosis and early treatment can prevent damage to vital organs.

FURTHER READING

1. Duggal, Lalit & Jain, Neeraj & Singh, Bhandari & Patel, Jeet & Goyal, Vishal & Gupta, Disha. (2021). IgG4-related disease: a review with an Indian perspective. International Journal of Research in Medical Sciences. 9. 2877. 10.18203/2320-6012.ijrms20213436.

2. Dua, A., Jain, N., Duggal, L., Chintala, B. (2022). Biologics in IgG4-Related Disease. In: Jain, N., Duggal, L. (Eds) Handbook of Biologics for Rheumatological Disorders. Springer, Singapore. https://doi.org/10.1007/978-981-16-7200-2_23

3. Stone J, Zen Y, Deshpande V. IgG4-related disease. N Engl J Med. 2012; 366(6):539–51.

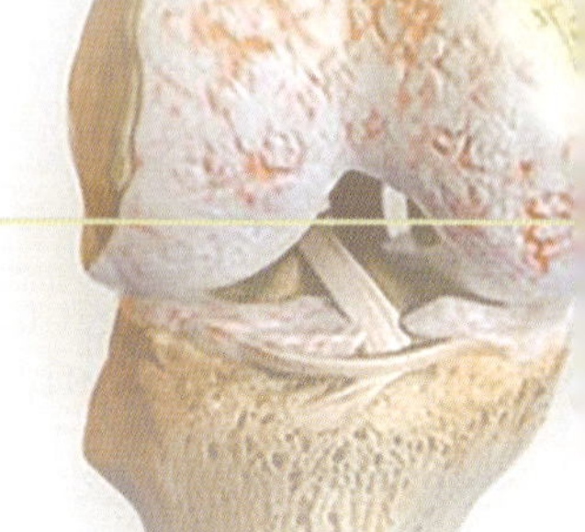

Adult-onset Still's Disease

Mohit Goyal

INTRODUCTION

Adult-onset Still's disease (AOSD) is a rare, complex, systemic, inflammatory disorder marked by high-grade, quotidian fever, polyarthritis, and a transient, salmon pink-coloured, maculopapular rash. In 1897, British physician George Still first documented a systemic onset juvenile arthritis that was named Still's disease. The adult variant offers different challenges and has a more severe presentation. AOSD is often not a straightforward diagnosis due to its heterogeneous presentation and lack of specific laboratory markers. The aetiology is not known. It has been thought to be a reactive syndrome triggered in response to infections in genetically predisposed individuals. There appears to be a slight predilection for women over men. Concerning age, AOSD has bimodal peaks, around 15–25 years and 35–45 years of age.

Clinical Features

The course of AOSD may be monophasic or intermittent and may evolve into chronic where it is predominantly articular. The three typical features of AOSD are:

- Fever is usually high grade, often intermittent, with fluctuations and complete defervescence may not occur in about a fifth of patients.
- Rash in AOSD is salmon-coloured, evanescent, macular or maculopapular and appears on the trunk and extremities. It is characteristically non-pruritic and usually comes and goes away with the fever.
- Arthritis often starts as mild and oligoarticular, but may progress to a severe, disabling polyarthritis. Knees, wrists, and ankles are most commonly involved and fusion of the wrist is characteristic. Other joints such as elbows, proximal interphalangeal joints, shoulders, metacarpophalangeal, metatarsophalangeal, hips, distal interphalangeal, and temporomandibular joints can also be involved.
- Other non-typical clinical features include fatigue, myalgia, pleuritis, pericarditis, hepatosplenomegaly, non-suppurative pharyngitis and lymphadenopathy. Uncommonly macrophage activation syndrome can occur.

Diagnosis

- The diagnosis of AOSD is based on the clinical picture aided by certain supportive laboratory findings. No test is pathognomonic of the condition.

- Serum ferritin level is a useful marker that is often raised more than five times the upper limit of normal. The test when used alone has high sensitivity and low specificity, but when combined with a concurrent fall in the proportion of glycosylated ferritin to less than 20%, the specificity increases to over 90%.
- Raised acute phase reactants (erythrocyte sedimentation rate and c-reactive protein), neutrophilic leukocytosis and thrombocytosis are seen in nearly all patients but are not specific. A normocytic normochromic anemia can occur. Elevated liver transaminases, aldolase and low positive titres of antinuclear antibodies and rheumatoid factor may be found.
- Synovial fluid is inflammatory and in those with longer disease durations, joint space narrowing, periarticular osteopenia and ankylosis of joints may be seen on conventional radiography.
- Computed tomography and fluorodeoxyglucose positron emission tomography can be useful to detect lymphadenopathy and organomegaly.

Diagnostic Criteria

The Yamaguchi criteria are commonly used to diagnose AOSD in adults.

Major Criteria

- Fever of at least 39°C lasting at least one week
- Arthralgias or arthritis lasting two weeks or longer
- A nonpruritic macular or maculopapular skin rash that is salmon-coloured in appearance and usually found over the trunk or extremities during febrile episodes
- Leukocytosis (10,000/mL or greater), with at least 80 percent granulocytes

Minor Criteria

- Sore throat
- Lymphadenopathy
- Hepatomegaly or splenomegaly
- Abnormal liver function studies, particularly elevations in aspartate and alanine aminotransferase and lactate dehydrogenase concentrations
- Negative tests for antinuclear antibody and rheumatoid factor

These criteria require the **presence of five features, with at least two being major** diagnostic criteria.

Treatment

The management of AOSD is targeted towards the control of symptoms, and prevention of deformities and other complications while minimizing the therapy related adverse effects. Response to treatment is assessed by reductions in serum ferritin level, erythrocyte sedimentation rate, C-reactive protein level and resolution of symptoms.

Glucocorticoids are often deployed at diagnosis and monotherapy is effective in many cases. However, to minimise the accrual of side effects the dose and duration are kept to the least required and other agents are added early. Response is usually inadequate to non-steroidal anti-inflammatory agents alone except in those with mild symptoms.

Interleukin-1 blockade by agents such as anakinra is effective and is deployed early, as the first line in severe, rapidly progressive disease after ruling out the possibility

Table 33.1: Current treatment options for adult-onset Still's disease		
Drug	*Dose*	*Notes*
Glucocorticoids	20–60 mg (prednisolone equivalent)	Effective as monotherapy. Steroid-sparing should be started early
Anakinra	100 mg once to twice a day subcutaneous	First choice in severe, rapidly progressive disease
Tocilizumab	4–8 mg/kg every 4 weeks	Used in glucocorticoid-resistant disease
Methotrexate	10–25 mg per week	Effective in arthritis but not systemic symptoms
Cyclosporin A	2.5–4 mg/kg per day	May be used in combination with methotrexate for systemic involvement
Non-steroidal anti-inflammatory drugs	Naproxen 500 mg twice daily Indomethacin 25 to 50 mg 3 times daily ibuprofen 800 mg 3 times daily	Effective as monotherapy in only mild disease

of sepsis. Interleukin-6 blockade with tocilizumab is another option in glucocorticoid-resistant disease. Methotrexate is effective in arthritis but has not been found to help in other systemic features. Cyclosporin A has been used for systemic involvement and there are reports of successful treatment of severe AOSD by combining it with methotrexate. Tumor necrosis factor blockade may be used in those with persistent arthritis without systemic symptoms. Treatment options are summarised in Table 33.1.

Prognosis

AOSD may be self-limiting, remain intermittent or evolve into chronic arthritis predominant disease. Severe polyarthritis at onset and resistant symptoms are poor prognostic markers.

Clinical Snippet

A 35-year-old woman presented with a 2-week history of fever, joint pain, and a rash. She had been previously diagnosed with seronegative rheumatoid arthritis and was taking methotrexate. However, her symptoms worsened, and she developed a new salmon pink rash. Upon further evaluation, it was discovered that her ferritin level was markedly elevated. Rheumatoid factor and antinuclear antibody tests were negative. A diagnosis of AOSD was made, and glucocorticoids were started, which led to a rapid improvement in her symptoms.

FURTHER READING

1. Bhargava J, Panginikkod S. Still Disease. [Updated 2024 Feb 26]. In: StatPearls [Internet]. Treasure Island (FL): StatPearls Publishing; 2024 Jan-. Available from: https://www.ncbi.nlm.nih.gov/books/NBK538345.

2. Leavis HL, van Daele PLA, Mulders-Manders C, Michels R, Rutgers A, Legger E, et al. Management of adult-onset Still's disease: evidence- and consensus-based recommendations by experts. Rheumatology (Oxford). 2024;63(6):1656–63.

Macrophage Activation Syndrome

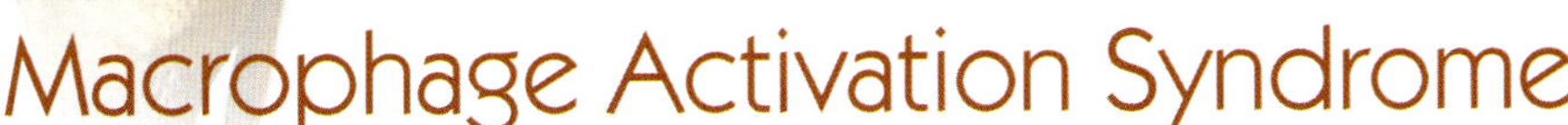

Himanshi Chaudhary, Pravin Patil

INTRODUCTION

Macrophage activation syndrome (MAS) is a severe and potentially life-threatening complication of rheumatological diseases. It is marked by improper activation of phagocytes, particularly macrophages and cytotoxic T cells. This leads to a cytokine storm, which triggers hemophagocytosis and causes damage to multiple organs. The most common autoimmune diseases associated with MAS are systemic juvenile idiopathic arthritis (SJIA), adult onset Still's disease(AOSD) followed by systemic lupus erythematosus (SLE), Kawasaki disease (KD), and juvenile dermatomyositis (JDM).[1] Coupled with its mimicry with other conditions, this goes unrecognized at times and can lead rapidly to critical illness and death. The estimated prevalence of MAS in SJIA was ~10%[2] and it has been reported in 5–19.5% patients with AOSD.[3] The prevalence in SLE varied from 0.9 to 4.6%,[4] and in KD ~1.3%.[5]

Clinical Features

Macrophage activation syndrome is a clinical syndrome which has symptoms and signs that overlap with and resemble those of other systemic illnesses, including sepsis, malignancy, and rheumatic diseases. Some diagnostic criteria involving clinical and laboratory data are available for defining MAS.[6–9] However, the relative changes in the clinical and laboratory features from baseline are more useful for providing an early diagnosis. Some of the important clinical findings are as follow:

1. Fever is universally seen in patients with MAS. Fever is typically non-remitting and high-grade. Persistent fever in unwell adults without an attributable cause, or worsening fever in patients with treated infection, should prompt investigation for MAS.
2. Hepatosplenomegaly can be seen in patients with an active disease.
3. Neurological symptoms like seizures, alterations in mental status, lethargy and headache can be seen in one-third of patients with MAS.[10]
4. Liver dysfunction and hemorrhagic manifestations can be seen in 20% of patients.
5. Severe cases may even result in heart, lung and kidney involvement, leading to a fatal outcome.[11]

Laboratory alterations include cytopenia, hypofibrinogenemia, elevated ferritin, lactate dehydrogenase, triglycerides, D-dimers and liver enzymes.

1. A fall in erythrocyte sedimentation rate in a febrile patient with high C-reactive protein should raise a suspicion of MAS.
2. Hemophagocytosis in bone marrow and tissues is a late feature of MAS and is not an essential criterion for classification of MAS.[7]
3. Specific serum markers of HLH include soluble CD25 and soluble CD163 reflect levels of T cell activation and degree of hemophagocytosis in patient with MAS.[12]
4. Serum ferritin levels closely mirror disease activity and serial ferritin measurement is useful for monitoring response to therapy. Ferritin levels >10 000 mg/L are 96% specific and 90% sensitive for HLH in children, although other criteria need to be met to make the diagnosis.[11] Ferritin levels are also closely related to disease activity and serial ferritin measurement is done to assess response to treatment.[13]

Diagnosis

The histiocyte society presented a set of diagnostic guidelines and treatment protocol for hemophagocytic lymphohistiocytosis (HLH) in 2004 that have traditionally been considered a scientific cornerstone for the diagnosis of HLH and MAS.[7] The details of the criteria are mentioned in Box 34.1. These criteria were primarily validated on patients less than 18 years of age. We know that triggers, organ reserve, fitness, and clinical presentation may differ between the pediatric and adult age groups, therefore, a revision of the recommendations were published by the histiocyte society in 2019.[9] Treatment with DMARDs, particularly biologics, can alter the clinical features of MAS, potentially limiting the effectiveness of established clinical criteria for diagnosing MAS. Patients receiving IL-1 and IL-6 blockers may experience lower ferritin levels, less pronounced drops in cell counts, and reduced fever spikes, yet they can still develop MAS.[14] It is, therefore, essential to evaluate the clinical status and trends in laboratory values over time to ensure that features of MAS are not overlooked, even if the clinical criteria are not fully met.

Box 34.1: HLH-2004 diagnostic guideline for HLH

Diagnosis of HLH can be established if one of the 2 criteria is fulfilled
1. Molecular diagnosis consistent with HLH
2. Diagnostic criteria fulfilled (5 out of the following fulfilled)
   a. Fever
   b. Splenomegaly
   c. Cytopenia (affecting ≥ 2 of 3 lineages in the peripheral blood): Hemoglobin <90 g/L, platelets <100 × 10^9/L, neutrophils <1.0 × 10^9/L
   d. Hypertriglyceridemia and/or hypofibrinogenemia: Fasting triglycerides 3.0 mmol/L (i.e., 265 mg/dl) fibrinogen 1.5 g/L
   e. Hemophagocytosis in bone marrow or spleen or lymph nodes
   f. No evidence of malignancy
   g. Ferritin 500 mg/L
   h. Soluble CD25 (i.e., soluble IL-2 receptor) 2,400 U/ml
   i. Low or absent NK-cell activity (according to local laboratory reference)

Treatment

There are no standard protocols for management of MAS in adults. The therapeutic plans have been extrapolated from treatment plans for familial HLH or MAS in SJIA. The HLH-2004 protocol described a combination chemotherapy of dexamethasone and etoposide along with cyclosporine and intrathecal methotrexate. This can be followed by a curative hematopoetic stem cell transplant in non-responders.[7] The 2019 modification of the criteria discussed that adults might not need a very aggressive chemotherapy regimen and considered adopting a more individualized and graded modification of HLH-2004 protocol.[9] Pulse methylprednisolone (1 gm/day for 3–5 consecutive days) and intravenous immunoglobulins (1–2 gm/kg) have been suggested as first line therapy in patients with non-organ threatening illness and etoposide may be considered in patients with severe HLH presenting with imminent organ failure.

In cases where patients do not respond adequately right away, cyclosporine (2–7 mg/kg per day) can be added to the treatment regimen. Additionally, IL-1-blocking therapy with anakinra is recommended, with suggested doses ranging from 2 to 6 mg/kg, up to a maximum of 10 mg/kg per day, administered subcutaneously in divided doses. Patients with residual disease after 8 weeks may benefit from maintenance therapy and, possibly, allogenic stem cell transplant. Parallel considerations include identification and treatment of triggers like infectious agents and malignancy in Table 34.1.

Prognosis

Expected disease course and outcomes: The prognosis of MAS depends on several factors, including underlying cause, time to diagnosis and treatment, severity of organ involvement and patient's overall health.

Without effective treatment, the mortality rate for patients with MAS is alarmingly high, ranging from 20 to 53%, and can reach up to 70% in certain cases.[11] Elevated serum ferritin levels have been linked to higher mortality, while a rapid decline in serum ferritin of more than 50% after treatment correlates with lower mortality rates. Additionally, older age at onset and the presence of comorbidities are associated with increased mortality.[12]

Physicians need to recognize the diverse presentations of MAS, particularly in the context of rheumatological conditions such as SJIA, AOSD, SLE, and pyrexia of unknown origin. Given the high morbidity and mortality rates, early identification is

Table 34.1: Drugs used in the treatment of MAS		
Drug Name	*Dose*	*Toxicity*
Intravenous Methylprednisolone	1 gm/day for 3–5 days	Hypertension, hyperglycemia, gastrointestinal bleeding, pancreatitis
Intravenous immunoglobulin	1–2 gm/kg	Infusion reactions, aseptic meningitis
Etoposide	150 mg/m^2 as per protocol	Myelosuppression, arrhythmia, hepatotoxicity
Cyclosporine	2–7 mg/kg/day	Hypertension, hyperglycemia, hepatotoxicity, nephrotoxicity
Anakinra	2–6 mg/kg/day	Injection site reactions, headaches, nasopharyngitis

vital for initiating prompt and aggressive treatment. Treatment strategy involves using combination immunosuppression and addressing co-triggers to achieve remission.

Clinical Snippet

A typical case of the disease with management: A 36-year-old lady who is a known case of SLE but has poor compliance to therapy has been having fever, joint pains and rashes since 2 months. The fever episodes have increased since 1 week and she also has pain abdomen and epistaxis. Examination reveals cervical lymphadenopathy and hepatosplenomegaly. Investigations show hemoglobin 5.6 g/dL, platelets 10,000/uL, total leucocyte count 1500/uL, ESR 10 mm/hr, CRP: 120 mg/dl, SGOT 256 U/L, SGPT 500 U/L, creatinine 1.1 mg/dl, INR: 2.1. Complements.

(C3,C4) are low and anti-dsDNA antibody levels are elevated. The high grade fever spikes, joint pains, rashes, cytopenia, transaminitis and elevated markers of disease activity make you think of disease activity, but the corresponding ESR/CRP mismatch and the new onset high grade fever spikes suggest a possibility of MAS. Serum ferritin is 8000 ng/ml, triglyceride levels are 280 mg/dl and fibrinogen 1.2 g/L further supporting a diagnosis of MAS in a patient with active SLE. A screening for infective agents like TB, EBV, CMV and malignancy is also done to look for triggers of MAS. She is treated with high dose methylprednisolone 1 gm/day for 3 days followed by oral high dose prednisolone. Blood parameters are repeated again after 3 days to look for clinical improvement. Based on clinical progression, further individualised therapeutic options are considered.

FURTHER READING

1. Ravelli A, Grom AA, Behrens EM, Cron RQ. Macrophage activation syndrome as part of systemic juvenile idiopathic arthritis: diagnosis, genetics, pathophysiology, and treatment. *Genes Immun.* 2012 Jun;13(4):289–98.
2. La Rosée P, Horne A, Hines M, Von Bahr Greenwood T, Machowicz R, Berliner N, et al. Recommendations for the management of hemophagocytic lymphohistiocytosis in adults. *Blood.* 2019 Jun 6;133(23):2465–77.
3. Minoia F, Davì S, Horne A, Demirkaya E, Bovis F, Li C, et al. Clinical features, treatment, and outcome of macrophage activation syndrome complicating systemic juvenile idiopathic arthritis: a multinational, multicenter study of 362 patients. *Arthritis Rheumatol.* 2014 Nov;66(11):3160–9.

Vasculitic Ulcers

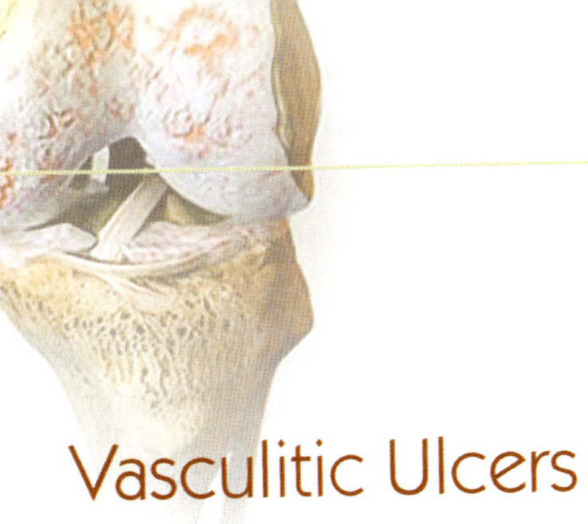

Pratyusha Rajavarapu

INTRODUCTION

Autoimmune rheumatic diseases (AIRD) can have many systemic manifestations and are known to affect any or all organ systems. Skin involvement is particularly very common in AIRDs and it can be of many different presentations. AIRD presenting as vasculitic ulcers is relatively less common but is usually associated with higher morbidity and mortality.

Normal wound healing involves 4 phases which are—hemostasis, inflammation, proliferation and remodeling. However, chronic wounds are arrested in the inflammatory phase and may result in upregulation of angiogenesis and matrix deposition. There are many etiologies for development of chronic non-healing wounds, the most common being occlusive vascular diseases. In a study done on 31,619 German patients, venous occlusion accounted for 47.6% followed by combined arterial and venous causes in 17.6% whereas arterial insufficiency accounted for 14.5%. Vasculitis accounted for 5.1% and pyoderma gangrenosum amounted to 3% of all the cases.

Vasculitic ulcers are usually the result of either small or medium vessel vasculitis. Vasculitis can be either primary systemic vasculitis or secondary to other systemic AIRDs. The common autoimmune diseases causing vasculitic ulcers include rheumatoid arthritis, scleroderma, mixed connective tissue disorders, ANCA associated vasculitis, systemic lupus erythematosus, pyoderma gangrenosum and so on. The severity and management depends on the type of underlying AIRD.

Vasculitic Ulcers in Different Rheumatic Conditions

1. **Rheumatoid arthritis:** It is one of the most common AIRDs associated with vasculitic leg ulcers. Ulcers in RA are associated with longer disease duration, higher rheumatoid factor titers and higher mortality. Felty's syndrome which is characterized by splenomegaly and neutropenia in a case of rheumatoid arthritis is also associated with skin ulcers. Whereas the development of ulcers is usually associated with disease activity, biopsy may be needed in certain cases for diagnosis and to rule out secondary infections. Treatment is aimed at both escalating the immunosuppressive therapy and restoring the blood flow. There is evidence of benefit in healing of vasculitic ulcers with biological DMARDs especially TNF inhibitors.

2. **Systemic sclerosis and MCTD:** Systemic sclerosis is a rare autoimmune disease characterized by immune activation, vasculopathy, fibroblast stimulation, and connective tissue fibrosis. MCTD is characterized by the presence of anti-RNP antibodies which may present with overlapping features of several AIRDs like SLE or RA. Lower extremity ulcers, a complication of long-standing scleroderma, affects about 4% of patients and is associated with significant morbidity. The etiology in scleroderma is often multifactorial but the most common histologic finding is fibrin occlusive vasculopathy with intimal thickening and some inflammation.

   Medical treatment options include vasodilators such as calcium channel blockers, prostanoids such as iloprost and endothelin receptor antagonists such as Bosentan. Topical and systemic opioids are often used to address the severe pain, but may delay the wound healing. Endovascular therapies have been tried but are not very effective owing to the presence of digital vasculopathy.

3. **ANCA associated vasculitis:** Primary systemic vasculitis is classified into large, medium and small vessel vasculitis depending upon the size of the affected vessel. Whereas large vessel vasculitis is associated with claudication pain or neurological manifestations, medium vessel vasculitis presents as digital ischemia or internal organ insufficiency symptoms. Small vessel vasculitis like ANCA associated vasculitis are more likely to be associated with vasculitic ulcers. All the three ANCA associated vasculitides, granulomatosis with polyangiitis (GPA, formerly known as Wegener's granulomatosis), microscopic polyangiitis (MPA), and the Churg-Strauss syndrome (CSS) have been associated with vasculitic leg ulcers.

   Pathologic findings included leukocytoclastic vasculitis with infiltration of arterioles and postcapillary venules by neutrophils undergoing degranulation and fragmentation with immunofluorescence showing complement deposits. Similar to ulcers caused by other AIRDs, aggressive treatment of the underlying autoimmune disease often results in healing of the wound. Anti-CD20 monoclonal antibodies like Rituximab have shown to be highly efficacious in treatment of ANCA vasculitis associated leg ulcers.

4. **SLE:** Vasculitic ulcers are rare complications of systemic lupus erythematosus and they are usually secondary to immune complex mediated vasculitis. In few patients, especially those who have secondary antiphospholipid antibodies histopathology may also show thrombo-occlusive findings. Though there are not many randomized control trials supporting the management of lupus related leg ulcers, it is proposed that aggressive immunosuppression in conjunction with steroids is needed.

5. **Pyoderma gangrenosum:** Pyoderma gangrenosum (PG) is a rare cutaneous predominant autoimmune condition characterized by development of a small pustule to begin with which later develops into a bulla and finally ulcerates. These lesions usually worsen with biopsy and surgery. PG can be associated with few systemic autoimmune diseases like inflammatory bowel disease, psoriasis, ankylosing spondylitis and few malignancies. Histopathologically PG is characterized by neutrophilic infiltration of dermis.

   Vasculitic ulcers can be associated with few other less common AIRDs like Sjögren's syndrome, cryoglobulinemia also.

FURTHER READING

1. Shanmugam V, DeMaria D, Attinger C. Lower extremity ulcers in rheumatoid arthritis: features and response to immunosuppression. Clinical Rheumatology. 2011; 30(6):849–53. [PubMed: 21340497]

2. Shanmugam V, Price P, Attinger C, Steen V. Lower Extremity Ulcers in Systemic Sclerosis: Features and Response to Therapy. Int J Rheumatol. 2010 pii:747946.

3. Dabiri G, Falanga V. Connective tissue ulcers. Journal of Tissue Viability. 2013; 22(4):92–102. [PubMed: 23756459]

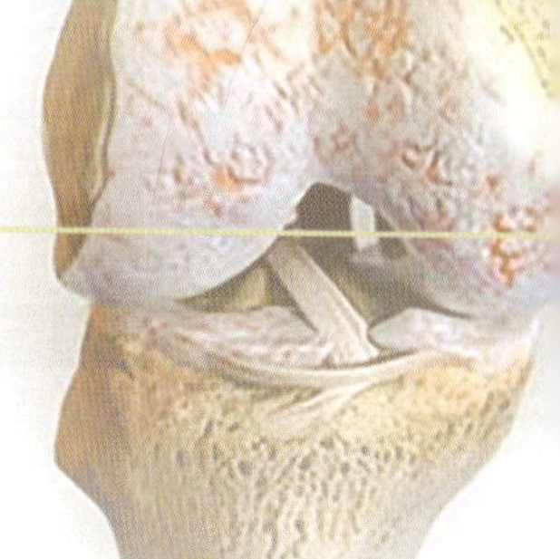

Pyoderma Gangrenosum

Sravan Kumar Appani

INTRODUCTION

Pyoderma gangrenosum (PG) was first described by Louis Brocq in 1908, and named by Brunsting et al in 1930 . PG is characterized by rapidly growing painful non healing, solitary ulcers with undermined borders and peripheral erythema. It falls into the category of neutrophilic dermatoses. PG is a misnomer as it is neither infectious nor gangrenous condition and it is a diagnosis of exclusion. These lesions are generally chronic, but can be relapsing and self-limiting.

PG is a rare disease with worldwide incidence of approximately 3–10 cases per million population per year. It most commonly affects middle aged females. Children are affected in 3–4 % cases. Exact pathophysiology is unclear. Neutrophil dysfunction, gene mutations, immune dysregulation (both adaptive and innate) play an important role in pathogenesis of PG . There is increased production of several pro-inflammatory chemokines and cytokines like IL-1, IL-6, IL-8, IL17 and IL-23. IL- 23 is important in activating neutrophils and stimulating IL-17 mediated inflammation Trauma induces release of IL-36 and IL-8 which play an important role in PG pathogenesis. Lesions show massive neutrophilic infiltration, haemorrhage, necrotic dermal vessels with no underlying infection or vasculitis. Main goal of biopsy is to exclude other diseases.

Clinical Features

Patients present with small red papule, pustule changing to deep ulcerative and granulomatous lesions with undermined edges and violaceous border that hangs over ulcer bed. These lesions heal by cribriform scar formation. Pain is the predominant complaint, arthralgias and malaise are often present. Five characteristics of PG include Painful, Progressive, Purple, Pretibial, Pathergy (exaggerated response to minor skin injury). Six clinical variants of PG include: ulcerative, bullous, pustular, vegetative, peristomal, and postoperative, few of them are discussed in Table 36.1. Most common extra cutaneous manifestation of PG is culture negative neutrophilic infiltrates involving lungs. Other organ systems include central nervous systems, gastrointestinal tract, eyes, liver, spleen, bones, lymph nodes.

Systemic associations: PG is often associated with systemic diseases in 25–50% cases, which include inflammatory bowel disease (Ulcerative colitis > Crohn's disease),

Table 36.1: Clinical variants of pyoderma gangrenosum

Variants	Clinical features	Site of Ulcer	Histopathology	Associated systemic illness
Ulcerative (Classical PG)	Necrotic ulcers with typical violaceous borders, granulation base	Sites of trauma, pretibial area	fibrin deposition, thrombosis, vascular damage, predominate neutrophilic infiltration	IBD, RA, seronegative arthritis, malignancies
Bullous	Painful vesicles coalesce to form bullae which, rapidly progress into ulcer	Face, upper limbs > lower limbs	Neutrophilic infiltration with microabscess, immunofluorescence is negative (rules out immunobullous diseases)	Lymphoproliferative diseases, IBD
Pustular	Sterile pustules with erythematous halo	Legs and abdomen	Subcorneal neutrophilic infiltration around hair follicles	IBD
Vegetative	Less painful, slow growing single ulcer, rapidly responds to therapy	Abdomen	Neutrophilic inflammation surrounded by histiocytes and lymphocytic infiltration	None

IBD: Inflammatory bowel disease; RA: Rheumatoid arthritis

rheumatoid arthritis, seronegative arthritis and hematological malignancies. Few syndromic presentations of PG in association with certain gene mutations are enlisted in Table 36.2.

Diagnostic Criteria

Heterogeneous and overlap presentation of PG poses challenges leading to diagnostic delay and misdiagnoses. Diagnosis is mainly based on clinical and histopathological features with exclusion of other differentials and there is no specific investigation. Two proposed criteria for PG diagnosis known as the Delphi consensus and the PARACELSUS score are detailed in Tables 36.3 and 36.4, respectively.

Differentials to consider for PG includes:
- Sweet syndrome (acute febrile neutrophilic dermatosis).
- Chronic venous and arterial insufficiency.
- Vasculitis.
- Traumatic ulceration, insect bites.
- Ulcerating infections, e.g. tuberculosis, blastomycosis, sporotrichosis.

Table 36.2: PG syndromic associations

PG syndromes	Clinical features	Associated genes
PAPA	PG, acne, pyogenic sterile arthritis	PSTPIP-1
SAPHO	Synovitis, acne, pustules, hyperostosis and osteitis	PSTPIP2, LPIN2, NOD2
PASH	PG, acne, hidradenitis suppurativa	MEFV, NOD2, NLRP3, PSMB8, NCSTN
PAPASH	PG, pyogenic arthritis, acne, hidradenitis suppurativa	PSTPIP1, IL1RN, MEFV

Table 36.3: The Delphi consensus criteria for the diagnosis of ulcerative PG (sensitivity 86%, specificity 90%)	
Major criterion (required)	Histopathology of ulcer edge must show a neutrophilic infiltrate.
Minor criteria (4 of 8 required)	1. Exclusion of infection 2. Pathergy 3. History of inflammatory bowel disease or inflammatory arthritis 4. History of papule, vesicle, or pustule ulcerating within four days 5. Peripheral erythema, undermining border, and tenderness at the ulcer site 6. Multiple ulcers, at least one on the anterior lower leg 7. Cribriform or wrinkled paper scars at the site of the healed ulcer 8. Decreased size of the ulcer within one month of initiating immunosuppressive medication.

Table 36.4: Paracelsus diagnostic score-score ≥10 is most likely PG	
Major criteria (3 points)	1. Progressive course of disease 2. Absence of relevant differential diagnosis 3. Reddish violaceous wound border
Minor criteria (2 points)	1. Responsive to immunosuppressive therapy 2. Irregular ulcer shape 3. Pain score >4/10 on visual analogue scale 4. Localised pathergy phenomenon
Additional criteria (1 point)	1. Undermined wound border 2. Suppurative inflammation in histopathology 3. Presence of systemic disease

- Squamous cell carcinoma, verrucous carcinoma.
- Ecthyma gangrenosum.
- Hidradenitis suppurativa.

Treatment

In patients with PG, it is important to treat the underlying systemic disease. Small ulcers are treated with topical steroids, tacrolimus ointment, intra-lesional steroid injections with regular dressings Oral prednisolone used as first line agent in severe disease. Oral prednisolone (0.5–1 mg/kg) and cyclosporine (3–5 mg/kg) used in severe disease have shown similar rate of ulcer healing 6 weeks post-initiation (STOP GAP randomised controlled trial). Steroid sparing agents' mycophenolate mofetil, dapsone, azathioprine, methotrexate, cyclophosphamide and intravenous immunoglobulins are used for moderate to severe PG. Therapies like anti-TNF alpha drugs-infliximab, etanercept, adalimumab, IL-12/23 inhibitor—Ustekinumab and jak inhibitors—tofacitinib have been successful in refractory cases. Wound care and pain control plays an important role in treatment of PG.

Prognosis

Prognosis of PG is unpredictable. Factors associated with poor prognosis include old age, bullous variants, secondary infection. Recurrence is seen in 30% and the mortality risk is three times higher than the general population.

FURTHER READING

1. Maverakis E, Ma C, Shinkai K, Fiorentino D, Callen JP, Wollina U, et al. Diagnostic criteria of ulcerative pyoderma gangrenosum: a delphi consensus of international experts. JAMA Dermatol 2018;154(4):461–6.
2. Jockenhöfer F, Wollina U, Salva KA, Benson S, Dissemond J. The PARACELSUS score: a novel diagnostic tool for pyoderma gangrenosum. Br J Dermatol 2019;180(3):615–20.
3. Ormerod AD, Thomas KS, Craig FE, Mitchell E, Greenlaw N, Norrie J, et al. Comparison of the two most commonly used treatments for pyoderma gangrenosum: results of the STOP GAP randomised controlled trial. BMJ 2015;350:h2958.

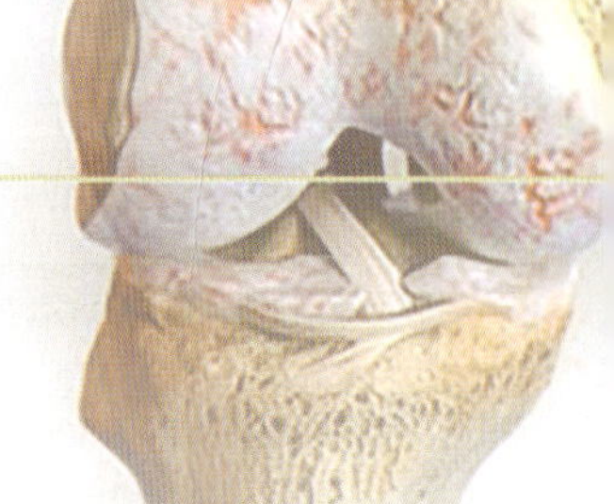

Erythema Nodosum

Saranya C

INTRODUCTION

Erythema nodosum (EN) was first described by Robert Willan in 1798. Erythema nodosum is the most common form of panniculitis, characterized by acute, painful, erythematous nodules or plaques, primarily affecting the subcutaneous fat. The condition is typically self-limited.

Epidemiology

- Demographics: Most commonly affects middle-aged women, particularly those aged 25–40 years.
- Gender ratio: Among adults, females are more frequently affected than males, with a ratio of 5:1. In children up to 12 years old, no significant sex difference is noted.

Etiology

EN can occur due to a vast number of underlying causes or associated conditions. In about 30–50% of cases, the cause is idiopathic, where no known aetiology can be identified. The possible causative or associated conditions are depicted in Table 37.1.

Pathogenesis

Erythema nodosum is thought to arise from a hypersensitivity reaction to various antigenic stimuli. These antigenic stimuli lead to the formation of immune complexes that deposit in the venules of subcutaneous fat. Some studies support the pathogenic role of these immune complexes and complement in causing tissue injury, while others have questioned this. Increased expression of adhesion molecules (e.g., P-selectin, E-selectin, platelet endothelial cell adhesion molecule, vascular cell adhesion molecule-1, and intercellular adhesion molecule-1) on endothelial cells has been observed. In addition, elevated levels of various inflammatory mediators (such as IL-6, IL-8, IL-12, interferon-γ, granulocyte colony-stimulating factor, monocyte chemoattractant protein-1, and tumor necrosis factor-α) have been detected in serum and skin samples. These inflammatory mediators recruit neutrophils, leading to neutrophilic inflammation, the production of reactive oxygen species, and subsequent tissue injury.

Table 37.1: Etiological factors of erythema nodosum	
Infections	**Drugs**
Bacterial	• Penicillin
• Streptococcal	• Sulphonamides
• Tuberculosis	• Oral contraceptive pills
• Leprosy	• Bromides
• Yersinia	• Iodides
• Mycoplasma	• TNF alpha blockers
• Bartonella	• Thalidomide
• Brucella	• Propylthiouracil
• Leptospirosis	• Isotretinoin
• Chlamydia	• Leukotriene modifiers
• Tularemia	• Hepatitis B vaccine
Viral	
• Infectious mononucleosis	
• Hepatitis B, C	
• HIV	
• HSV	
• EBV	
Fungal	
• Histoplasmosis	
• Blastomycosis	
• Coccidioidomycosis	
Parasitic	
• Amoebiasis	
• Giardiasis	
Systemic diseases	**Miscellaneous**
• Sarcoidosis	• Cutaneous T cell and other lymphomas
• Inflammatory bowel diseases	• Acute myeloid leukemia
• Systemic lupus erythematosus	• Pregnancy
• Dermatomyositis	
• Systemic sclerosis	
• Sweet syndrome	
• Behcet's disease	

Clinical Presentation

Patients with erythema nodosum typically present with:
- **Skin lesions:** Acute onset of one or more painful, erythematous, firm nodules or plaques, measuring 1–6 cm in diameter, primarily located on the extensor surfaces of the lower extremities.
- **Distribution:** Lesions are often bilateral and symmetrical. Occasionally, they may appear on the ankles, thighs, forearms, and trunk.
- **Prodromal symptoms:** In some patients, prodromal symptoms like fever, malaise, and/or arthralgia often precedes the skin lesions.
- **Systemic symptoms:** Additional symptoms can include headache, vomiting, abdominal pain, diarrhea, weight loss, and lymphadenopathy.

- **Evolution of lesions:** As the lesions develop, they may become more ecchymotic and typically heal within 4–6 weeks without resulting in atrophy, ulceration, or scar formation.

Diagnosis

- **Clinical presentation:** Diagnosis is primarily based on the characteristic clinical features.
- **Skin biopsy:** Either deep incisional or excisional biopsy including subcutaneous fat is performed to confirm the diagnosis.
- **Histological findings:**
  - *Septal panniculitis:* The biopsy shows characteristic septal panniculitis with a mixed cellular infiltrate, including lymphocytes, histiocytes, giant cells, and occasional eosinophils, without evidence of associated vasculitis.
  - *Miescher's radial granulomas:* These consist of a small collection of histiocytes arranged around a central star-shaped cleft, representing a relatively specific, but not pathognomonic, finding. Small and medium-sized vasculitis has been reported occasionally.
- Meticulous history taking and detailed physical examination are crucial for identifying potential underlying causes.
- The initial workup includes complete blood count, inflammatory markers (erythrocyte sedimentation rate, C-reactive protein), anti-streptolysin O titer, throat swab culture and chest radiography.
- Investigations like sputum AFB, tuberculin skin test, mycobacterial cultures and interferon release assays are performed in tuberculosis endemic regions.
- If initial evaluations do not yield conclusive results, additional imaging and laboratory tests may be needed to explore underlying systemic causes.
- Differential diagnosis of EN is depicted in Box 37.1.

Box 37.1: Differential diagnosis of EN

- Superficial thrombophlebitis
- Cutaneous polyarteritis nodosa
- Lupus panniculitis
- Erythema induratum of bazin
- Erythema nodosumleprosum
- Pancreatic panniculitis
- Panniculitis-like T cell lymphoma
- Alpha-1 antitrypsin deficiency

Management

In patients with erythema nodosum, secondary to systemic diseases, it is crucial to manage the underlying condition. While the majority of idiopathic EN is self-limiting, some patients may require symptomatic treatment for the management of pain.

Symptomatic Treatment

- **Analgesics:** Nonsteroidal anti-inflammatory drugs (e.g., ibuprofen, naproxen) are typically the first line for pain relief and to reduce inflammation.
- **Other options:** Colchicine has been used especially in EN associated with Behcet's disease. Systemic corticosteroids may be used in selected cases to reduce inflammation. An underlying infection or malignancy should be ruled out before considering steroid therapy.

- **Supportive measures:**
  - Compression bandages
  - Limb elevation
  - Bed rest to alleviate edema and discomfort.

Refractory or Recalcitrant Cases

- For lesions that do not respond to standard treatment, additional therapies may be considered:
  - Dapsone
  - Hydroxychloroquine
  - Oral potassium iodide
  - Intralesional steroids
  - Tetracyclines
  - Thalidomide
  - Cyclosporine
  - Tumor necrosis factor—inhibitors

Prognosis

The prognosis for erythema nodosum is generally excellent, with most patients experiencing spontaneous complete resolution of lesions within a few weeks.

FURTHER READING

1. De Simone C, Caldarola G, Scaldaferri F, Petito V, Perino F, Arena V, et al. Clinical, histopathological, and immunological evaluation of a series of patients with erythema nodosum. Int J Dermatol. 2016;55 (5):e289–e294.
2. Pérez-Garza DM, Chavez-Alvarez S, Ocampo-Candiani J, Gomez-Flores M. Erythema Nodosum: A Practical Approach and Diagnostic Algorithm. Am J Clin Dermatol. 2021;22(3):367–78.

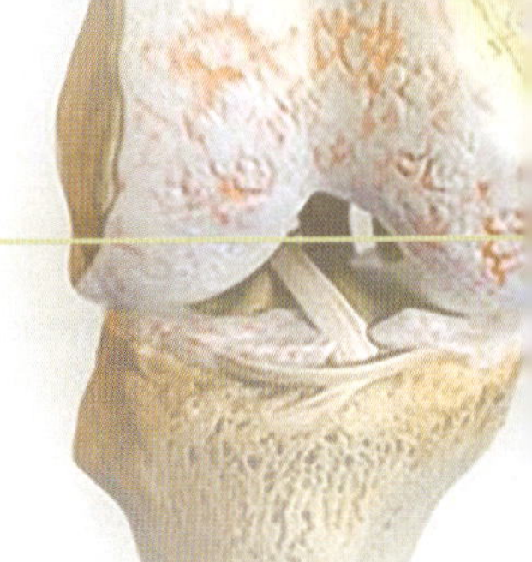

Raynaud's Disease

Amirtha Gopalan

INTRODUCTION

Raynaud phenomenon is a transient and peripheral vasoconstrictive response to cold temperatures or emotional stress. It was first described by French physician Maurice Raynaud in 1862. It is prevalent in 3–5% of the general population. Patients with raynaud's phenomenon are classified into two groups; those with primary Raynaud's phenomenon, which is diagnosed when no underlying disease is found; and those with secondary Raynaud's phenomenon, which is diagnosed when there is associated disease.

Clinical Features

Raynaud phenomenon typically affect fingers (distal areas). Attack starts out with a single digit and then spreads to other digits symmetrically on both hands. The thumb is typically spared. It may also result in cutaneous vasospasm affecting facial areas, ears, knees, or nipples. Raynaud's phenomenon is classically described with a triphasic colour change of the digits

1. Initial white or pallor (ischemic phase),
2. Blue or cyanosis (deoxygenation phase),
3. Followed by red or erythema (reperfusion phase).

Attacks are triggered by exposure to a cold environment, emotional stress, or from other physical or medication exposures. A typical attack may last less than an hour but can also persist for hours. As a result of vasoconstriction, pin and needles sensation, numbness or finger aches or pain are common complaints with Raynaud phenomenon attacks.

Clues that may raise concern for secondary Raynaud's include age of onset greater than age 40, male gender, digital ulcerations, asymmetric attacks, ischemic signs proximal to the fingers and toes, and abnormal nailfold capillaroscopy.

Feature	Primary Raynaud's phenomenon	Secondary Raynaud's phenomenon
Age at onset	Younger (15–20 years)	Older (30 years)
Prevalence	Common	Rare
Family history	Yes	No
Severity	Mild	Moderate to severe

(Contd.)

(Contd.)

Feature	Primary Raynaud's phenomenon	Secondary Raynaud's phenomenon
Associated with rheumatic disease	No	Yes
ANA positive	None to low titre ANA	Yes
Secondary changes	No	Digital ulcers, scars, gangrene, livedo reticularis
Nail fold capillaroscopy	Normal capillaries	Giant capillaries, drop outs, hemorrhages

Disease Associations

1. **Connective tissue disorders:** Scleroderma, lupus, or mixed connective tissue disease.
2. **Drug-induced:** Ergot, beta-blockers, dextroamphetamine, bleomycin, cisplatin, clonidine, cocaine, cyclosporine, interferon-alpha, nicotine, and vinblastine
3. **Endocrine causes:** Pheochromocytoma, carcinoid syndrome, or thyroid disease.
4. **Structural causes:** Thoracic outlet syndrome, atherosclerosis, brachiocephalic trunk disease as in Takayasu's arteritis, Buerger's disease or thromboangiitis obliterans cold injury.
5. **Hematologic causes:** Cryoglobulinemia, cryofibrinogenemia, paraproteinemia, or polycythemia.

Mimickers of Raynaud's include other vascular disorders such as acrocyanosis and erythromelalgia.

Treatment

Patient education is the primary therapy recommended. Avoiding sudden cold and rapid changes in temperatures should be emphasised. Patients should be counselled to avoid tobacco and caffeine which may exacerbate symptoms. Patients with primary Raynaud's usually do not need drug treatment. Pharmacologic therapy is advised for secondary forms of Raynaud's according to severity of episodes.

- **First line for mild to moderate events:** Calcium channel blockers like nifedipine or amlodipine
- **Severe events with digital ulcers/gangrene:** Phosphodiesterase 5 blockers, anti-platelets, statins, endothelin receptor antagonists (for Raynaud's associated with scleroderma)
- **Refractory cases:** Prostacyclins, digital sympathectomy

Referral to a rheumatologist is recommended to help evaluate for an underlying rheumatologic condition and to guide future therapy.

Outcomes

The prognosis for patients with primary Raynaud phenomenon in young people is good with little morbidity or mortality. However, patients with secondary Raynaud's can have severe, refractory or relapsing episodes leading to poor quality of life.

FURTHER READING

1. Temprano KK. A Review of Raynaud's Disease. Mo Med. 2016 Mar-Apr;113(2):123-6. PMID: 27311222; PMCID: PMC6139949.
2. Hochberg Textbook of Rheumatology, 8th Edition.

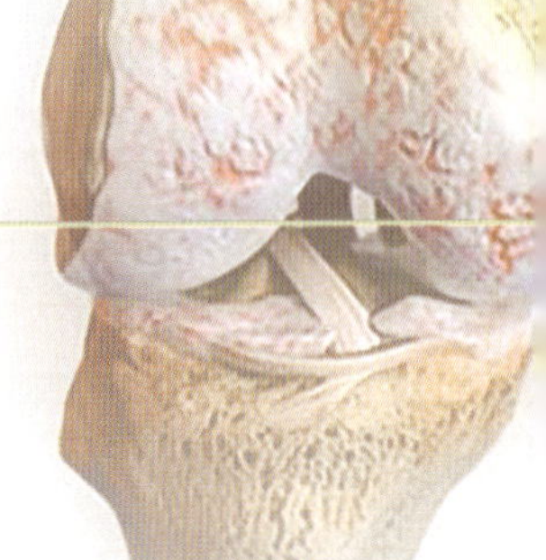

Pemphigus Vulgaris

Deepika Ponnuru

INTRODUCTION

Pemphigus belongs to autoimmune blistering disorders of skin, which is characterized by '*Acantholysis*' (loss of cell-cell adhesion) leading to blister formation within the epidermis of skin and the mucosa close to it. It is mediated by IgG antibodies against desmoglein-1(DSG1) and desmoglein-3(DSG3), which are structural components of desmosomes that play a pivotal role in cell-cell adhesion and maintain structural integrity of stratified squamous epithelium.

Three major subtypes of pemphigus include Pemphigus vulgaris, pemphigus foliaceus and paraneoplastic pemphigus in Table 39.1.

The clinical presentation of pemphigus varies based on the distribution of desmogleins in the epidermis, with DSG1 predominant in superficial skin layers and DSG3 in basal layers and mucous membranes, influenced by genetic predisposition and environmental triggers.

Clinical Features

- Common between ages 30 and 60, more frequent in women. The mucocutaneous variant starts with oral mucosal blisters, often flaccid and easily ruptured, leading to painful erosions, malnutrition, and weight loss. Other sites include conjunctiva, larynx, esophagus, nose, genitalia, and anus.

Table 39.1: Common subtypes of pemphigus and their clinical characteristics	
Pemphigus vulgaris	• Most common and life threatening condition if left untreated • 3 subtypes—mucocutaneous,mucosal and cutaneous forms • Anti DSG3 and anti-DSG1 antibodies are elevated-mucocutaneous is commonest
Pemphigus foliaceus	• Very superficial blisters/erosions. • No mucosal involvement • Anti DSG1 antibodies are specific • Good prognosis
Paraneoplastic pemphigus	• Common in elderly • Severe painful mucosal ulcers-refractory to treatment • Associated with malignancy, Grave prognosis • Anti DSG1,anti DSG3, antibodies to desmocollins, plakins

- **Skin lesions:** Flaccid blisters, erosions, and crusting on erythematous or normal skin, mainly on the head, upper trunk, and groin. Lesions are polymorphic and may show a positive Nikolsky sign, indicating fragile cell adhesion.

Diagnosis

The diagnosis of pemphigus is based on clinical history and histopathological findings supported by either direct immunofluorescence (DIF) or specific antibodies by ELISA/ indirect immunofluorescence.

- **Histopathology:** Gold standard for diagnosis. Lesional and perilesional biopsies from fresh blisters (<24 hours) show acantholysis and intraepidermal blister formation. Pemphigus foliaceus shows superficial blisters, while pemphigus vulgaris shows deep suprabasal blisters with a 'tombstone effect.'
- **DIF:** Performed on perilesional skin (1 cm from blister) to detect IgG and C3 deposits, showing a honeycomb or fish-net appearance. Paraneoplastic pemphigus shows additional dermoepidermal junction deposits.
- **Serology:** ELISA detects antidesmoglein antibodies, correlating with disease activity and useful for monitoring.

Treatment

Primary goal of treatment is to control the disease activity (existing lesions begin to heal and no new lesions form) and then complete remission (absence of new and existing lesions while on minimal therapy), i.e, remission induction (80% of lesions heal and no new lesions form over the past 2 weeks) and remission maintenance similar to other systemic autoimmune diseases.

Management of pemphigus vulgaris depends on the extent of involvement. Corticosteroids and rituximab (FDA approved) remain the mainstay of initial treatment. Other first line agents are mycophenolate mofetil and azathioprine while methotrexate, cyclophosphamide, cyclosporine are considered as second line agents in refractory cases.

Clinical Snippet

A 22 years old male presented with blistering skin lesions over the scalp and shoulders, and oral ulcers for 6 months. He was treated elsewhere with oral steroids at varying doses, with which lesions healed but recurred. The lesions had progressed rapidly over the last 10 days involving oral cavity, face, scalp, chest, abdomen, back and groin (Fig. 39.2). Blisters ruptured leaving large ulcers. Nikolsky's sign was positive. He was initiated on 1mg/kg oral prednisolone along with mycophenolate mofetil (MMF)- no response and had been developing new lesions. Then he received intravenous

Table 39.2: Other bullous disorders	
Autoimmune diseases	Bullous pemphygoid, lichen planus pemphigoides, SLE, IgA dermatosis, etc.
Infections	Staphylococcal scalded skin syndrome, herpetic stomatitis, bullous impetigo
Genetic	Hailey-Hailey disease
Others	Stevens-Johnson syndrome, toxic epidermal necrolysis, erythema multiforme, graft versus host disease, Grover disease, Seborrheic dermatosis, etc.

Table 39.3: List of medications effective in pemphigus vulgaris with possible adverse reactions			
Drug Name	Dose	Toxicity/Contraindications	Special Notes
Corticosteroids	0.5–1.5 mg/kg	Coexisting severe infections, uncontrolled diabetes mellitus	Intravenous pulse steroids are reserved for severe and refractory cases.
Rituximab	2 × 1000 mg IV-2 weeks apart or 375 mg/sqm every week for 4 weeks	Cytokine infusion reactions, infections	Recommended as first line steroid sparing immunosuppressive in new moderate to severe disease or refractory to other immunosuppressants.
Azathioprine	1–3 mg/kg/day	Leukopenia, transaminitis, DRESS	TPMT levels measurement to prevent serious bone marrow suppression
Mycophenolate mofetil	30–45 mg/kg/day	Contraindicated during coexisting severe infections	
IVIG	2 grams/kg over 2–5 days per month	Relatively safe during active coexisting infection. Contraindicated in renal failure	IgA deficient individuals should receive IgA depleted IVIG
Cyclophosphamide	1–2 mg/kg oral or 500–750 mg IV monthly	Infections, bone marrow suppression, long term risk of bladder carcinoma	Reserved as second line adjuvant immunosuppressant in refractory cases
Immunoadsorption	First line in emergency situations, if avaialble	Severe systemic infections, severe cardiovascular diseases,extensive hemorrhagic diathesis etc	Extracorporeal circuit is used to remove circulating antibodies and immune complexes by adsorption

TPMT: Thiopurine methyltransferase; IVIG: Intravenous immunoglobulins; DRESS: Drug reaction with eosinophilia and systemic symptoms

methylprednisolone (1 gram × 3 days) and rituximab (1 gram—2 weeks apart). His lesions started healing in a few days and attained complete remission within 1 month. Steroids were tapered and stopped in 2 months and maintained on MMF 1gram/day. One year later he developed new skin lesions which healed with 0.5 mg/kg prednisolone and MMF 2 grams/day. He is stable and is under regular follow up.

FURTHER READING

1. Malik AM, Tupchong S, Huang S, Are A, Hsu S, Motaparthi K. An Updated Review of Pemphigus Diseases. Medicina (Kaunas). 2021 Oct 9;57(10):1080. doi: 10.3390/medicina57101080. PMID: 34684117; PMCID: PMC8540565.
2. Zhao W, Wang J, Zhu H, Pan M. Comparison of Guidelines for Management of Pemphigus: a Review of Systemic Corticosteroids, Rituximab, and Other Immunosuppressive Therapies. Clin Rev Allergy Immunol. 2021 Dec;61(3):351-362. doi: 10.1007/s12016-021-08882-1. Epub 2021 Aug 4. PMID: 34350539.
3. Buonavoglia A, Leone P, Dammacco R, Di Lernia G, Petruzzi M, Bonamonte D, Vacca A, Racanelli V, Dammacco F. Pemphigus and mucous membrane pemphigoid: An update from diagnosis to therapy. Autoimmun Rev. 2019 Apr;18(4):349-358. doi: 10.1016/j.autrev.2019.02.005. Epub 2019 Feb 7. PMID: 30738958.

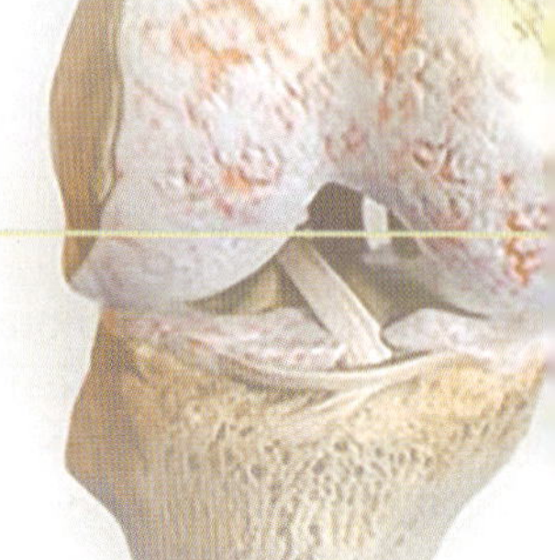

Renal Tubular Acidosis

Akshay Parikh

INTRODUCTION

The term "renal tubular acidosis" (RTA) refers to a group of disorders in which, despite a normal GFR, metabolic acidosis develops because the renal tubules are unable to maintain acid–base balance. All forms of RTA are characterized by a normal anion gap (hyperchloremic) metabolic acidosis.

Renal acid–Base Homeostasis

It is maintained by:

a. Proximal HCO_3^- reabsorption and
b. Distal urinary acidification

The text would be:

a. **HCO_3^- reabsorption in proximal convoluted tubule:** In the proximal tubule, H^+ ions are secreted into the lumen via the Na^+/H^+ exchanger (NHE-3), where they combine with filtered HCO_3^- to form carbonic acid (H_2CO_3). Luminal carbonic anhydrase IV (CA IV) catalyzes the breakdown of H_2CO_3 into CO_2 and H_2O, which diffuse into the tubular cells. Inside the cell, cytoplasmic carbonic anhydrase II (CA II) facilitates the recombination of CO_2 and H_2O into H_2CO_3, which dissociates into H_2 and HCO_3^-. The H^+ is recycled back into the lumen, while HCO_3^- is transported into the bloodstream via the sodium-bicarbonate cotransporter (NBC-1), ensuring efficient bicarbonate reabsorption.

b. **H^+ secretion in cortical collecting tubule:** In the cortical collecting tubule, intercalated cells are responsible for active H^+ secretion into the lumen via vacuolar H^+-ATPase and H^+,K^+-ATPase, which utilize ATP to pump H^+ ions against their gradient. This process acidifies the tubular fluid, facilitating the excretion of ammonium (NH_4^+) and titratable acids. Intracellularly, CA II catalyzes the formation of H_2CO_3 from CO_2 and H_2O, which dissociates into H^+ and HCO_3^-. The H^+ is secreted into the lumen, while HCO_3^- exits the cell into the bloodstream through the anion exchanger (AE1), which exchanges HCO_3^- for Cl^-. These complementary mechanisms in the proximal tubule and cortical collecting tubule ensure acid–base balance by reclaiming bicarbonate and excreting hydrogen ions.

Classification of RTA

There are three major forms of RTA which differ in their pathophysiology and clinical manifestations. Type 1 and 2 are hypokalemic while type 4 is hyperkalemic subtype.

- **Distal (type 1) RTA** is caused by defects in distal hydrogen ion excretion.
- **Proximal (type 2) RTA** is caused by defects in bicarbonate reabsorption in the proximal tubule. Some forms have generalized proximal tubule dysfunction called Fanconi syndrome.
- **Type 4 RTA** is caused by reductions in aldosterone secretion or responsiveness.

Clinical Manifestations of RTA

Manifestation	Normal kidneys	Proximal RTA	Distal RTA	Type 4 RTA
Urine pH	<5.2	Early stage >7 Late stage <5.2	**>5.5**	<5.2
Serum K^+	Normal	Low	Low	**High**
Osteomalacia	Absent	**Present***	**Present***	Absent
Nephrocalcinosis	Absent	Absent	**Present#**	Absent
Urine citrate	Normal	Normal	**Low**	Normal
Urine $NH4^+$	Normal	Low/Normal	Low	Low

*Osteomalacia occurs due to exchange of hydrogen ions for sodium, potassium, calcium, carbonate and phosphate in the bone. The continuous sequestration of protons in bone stimulates both osteoclast differentiation and osteoclast activity.

#The pathogenesis of nephrocalcinosis in distal RTA includes low urinary citrate, high urinary calcium, and high urinary pH favoring calcium phosphate precipitation.

RTA in Rheumatology

Primary Sjögren's Syndrome (pSS)

It is the most common acquired cause of distal RTA. Renal involvement in pSS has been reported in less than 10% of patients and is characterized by interstitial nephritis or, more rarely, glomerulonephritis. The interstitial nephritis may remain asymptomatic for a long period and may eventually present with features of distal RTA like hypokalemic paralysis, nephrocalcinosis, osteomalacia with bone pains and stress fractures. RTA can be the first manifestation of pSS.

Renal biopsy shows tubulointerstitial nephritis with lymphoplasmacytic infiltrate around the tubules with sparing of the glomeruli. Immunocytochemical analyses in few cases have shown complete absence of H^+-ATPase pumps in the intercalated cells. High titers of autoantibody directed against carbonic anhydrase II have also been identified in some patients.

Type 2 RTA can rarely occur in pSS. Occassionally it may be associated with urinary loss of phosphate, uric acid, glucose, amino acids and low molecular weight proteins as part of the Fanconi syndrome.

Systemic Lupus Erythematosus (SLE)

Interstitial involvement in the form of RTA has been rarely reported in SLE with most reports on type 1 RTA. Unlike pSS, it is frequently associated with significant proteinuria due to glomerulonephritis along with high ds-DNA antibody titres and low complement levels (C3 & C4). Hyperkalemic RTA has also been reported with SLE but not with pSS.

Diagnosis

Renal tubular acidosis (RTA) is diagnosed biochemically through arterial blood gas (ABG) analysis. Common electrolyte imbalances include hypo- or hyperkalemia. Osteomalacia may present with elevated alkaline phosphatase (ALP) and low serum calcium and phosphorus. X-rays can show diffuse osteopenia, stress fractures/Looser's zones/ pseudofractures. Stress fractures are typically transverse, do not span the entire width of bone, and are surrounded by localized periosteal reaction, commonly found in the scapula, subtrochanteric region, or pubic ramus (Fig. 40.1).

Treatment

Involvement limited to tubular acidosis without renal failure or glomerular involvement in pSS and SLE warrants only bicarbonate, potassium and calcium supplementation.

Sodium bicarbonate tablets	Starting dose	Goal
If serum bicarbonate <16 mEq/L	30 mEq four times daily (total 120 mEq)*	Titrate every week to attain 22–24 mEq/L of serum bicarbonate
If serum bicarbonate >16 mEq/L	40 mEq twice daily (total 80 mEq)*	
Potassium supplementation		
Syrup potassium citrate	As per potassium deficit	To correct hypokalemia[#]

*Note-1 gram of sodium bicarbonate tablet contains 12 mEq of bicarbonate.

[#]Correction of the metabolic acidosis with alkali therapy reduces inappropriate urinary potassium losses, which often corrects the associated hypokalemia. Thus reducing requirement of potassium supplementation over time.

Prognosis

RTA is a permanent disease. Prognosis is excellent if diagnosed early and appropriate supplements are continuously administered. Alkali therapy restores bone health and prevents the progression of nephrocalcinosis.

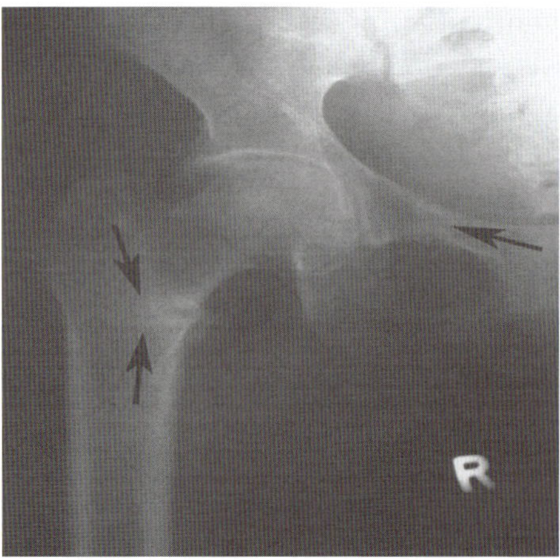

Fig 40.1: X-ray of right hip showing diffuse osteopenia and stress fracture in the superior pubic ramus (single arrow) and subtrochanteric femur (double arrows)

Clinical Snippet

A 30-year-old female presented with a year-long history of worsening pain in the right groin, ribs, and left shin, with inability to walk for the past month. She experienced multiple episodes of quadriparesis, each resolving with IV potassium. These episodes ceased after starting oral potassium citrate a year ago. Lab tests revealed normal anion gap metabolic acidosis (pH 7.22, HCO_3 16), low potassium (3.4), and elevated ALP (350), with X-ray showing a right hip stress fracture. Further investigation revealed sicca symptoms and positive anti-Ro/La antibodies, leading to a diagnosis of primary Sjögren's syndrome with distal renal tubular acidosis and osteomalacia. She was treated with sodium bicarbonate, calcium, vitamin D, and potassium, leading to significant improvement.

FURTHER READING

1. Chapter 147, Sjögren syndrome, Textbook of Rheumatology, Marc Hochberg, 8th edition.
2. EULAR recommendations for the management of Sjogren's syndrome with topical and systemic therapies, Ramos-Casals M, et al. Ann Rheum Dis 2020.

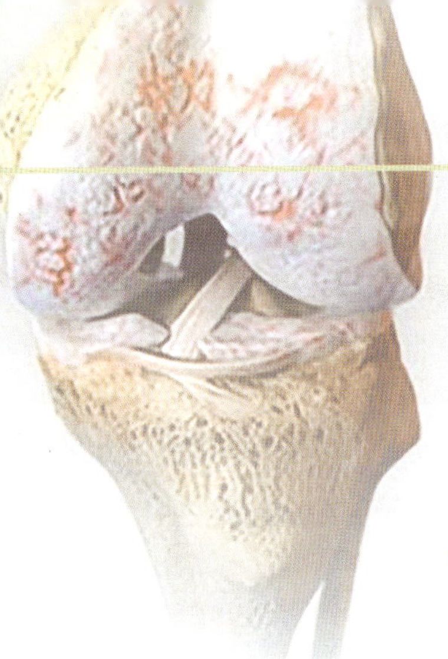

Vasculitides

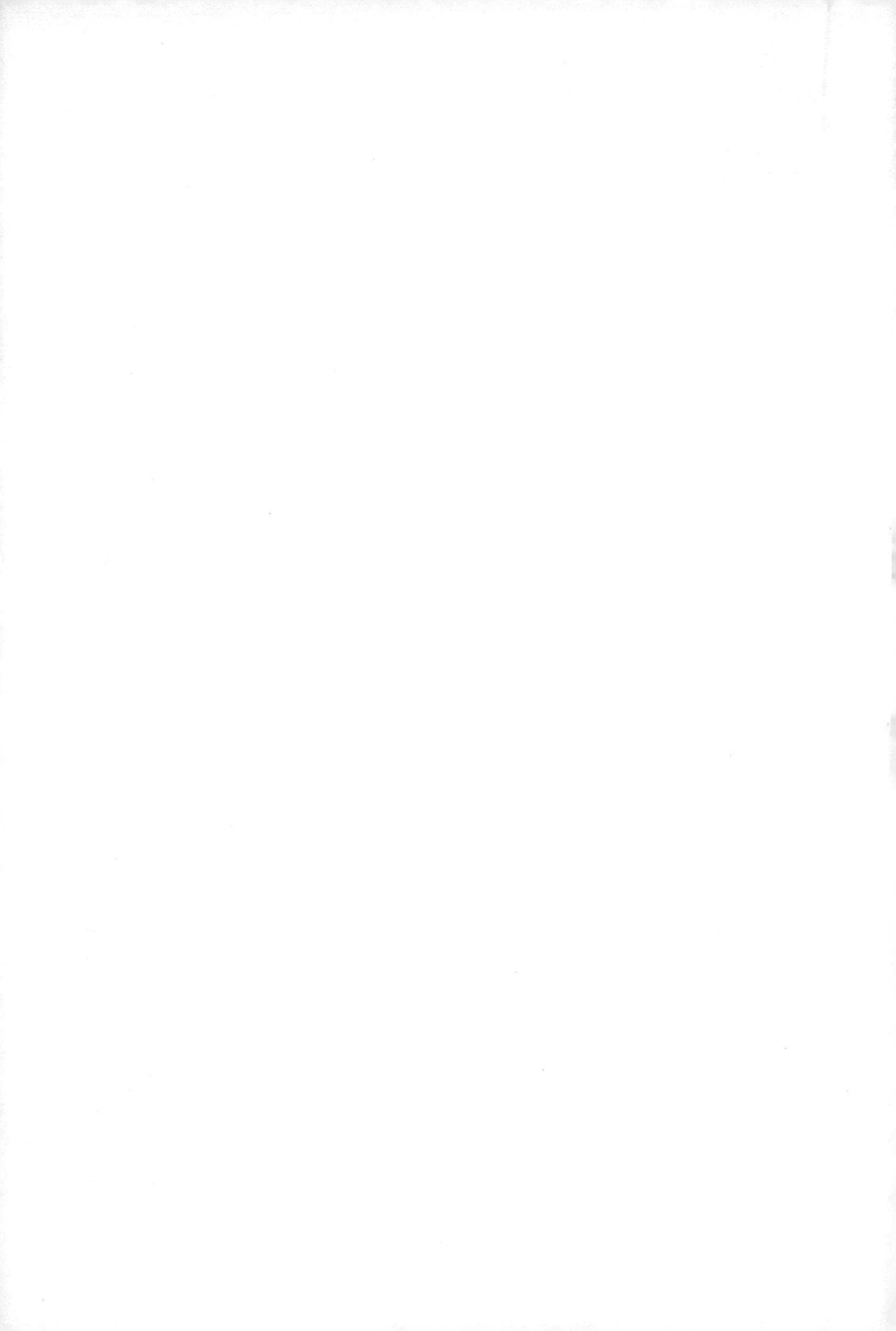

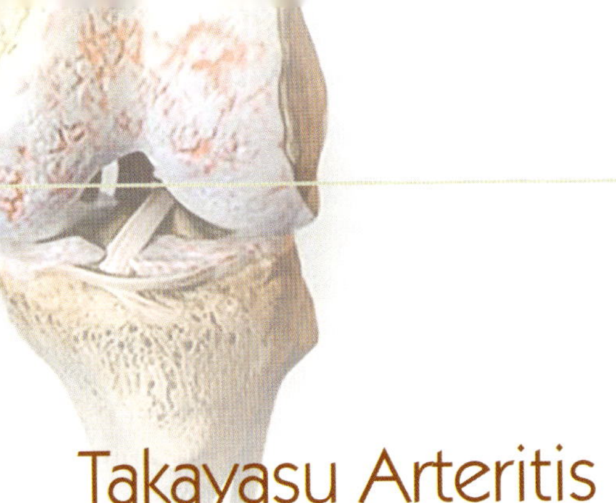

Takayasu Arteritis

Durga Prasanna Misra

INTRODUCTION

Takayasu arteritis (TAK) is a large vessel vasculitis (LVV) commonly seen in India, Southeast Asia, and South America. Granulomatous inflammation of the aorta and its major branches in TAK often results in stenosis of the affected arteries due to excessive arterial wall fibrosis. TAK more commonly affects young females

Clinical Features

The presentation of TAK is varied. Patients might be asymptomatic, and diagnosed with TAK when asymmetry of blood pressure, a missing peripheral pulse, or a vascular bruit is detected during clinical examination for another purpose. On the other hand, there might be prominent constitutional features such as fever, weight loss, and night sweats even when the patient has not yet developed any deficit of the peripheral pulses. There might be clinically evident arterial inflammation in the form of carotidynia (tenderness upon palpation of the carotid arteries). Renal artery stenosis or involvement of the descending thoracic or abdominal aorta (even without renal artery stenosis) can result in renovascular hypertension. Claudication of the upper or lower limbs can result from ischemia resulting from stenosis of the subclavian or common iliac arteries. Dilatation of the ascending aorta can result in aortic regurgitation. Critical organ ischemia of relatively rapid onset can result in ischemic stroke, myocardial infarction, or less commonly, ischemic optic neuropathy. Generally, arterial involvement in patients with TAK occurs over months to years, therefore, extensive collateral vessel formation can occur to restore arterial blood flow distal to the site of anatomical occlusion.

Diagnosis

Diagnostic criteria for TAK were proposed by Ishikawa in 1988 and later modified by Sharma and colleagues in 1996. Classification criteria for TAK were originally published from the American College of Rheumatology (ACR) in 1990. Later, data-driven criteria were published collaboratively by the ACR and the European Alliance of Associations for Rheumatology (EULAR) in 2022. It must be remembered that classification criteria are meant to homogenize recruitment in clinical trials involving patients with TAK and should not be used for clinical diagnosis.

In the appropriate clinical context (clinical features when present as described in the previous section), the diagnosis of TAK relies on angiography. Classically, conventional angiography was used but is not recommended nowadays unless the patient is planned for an endovascular intervention. Computed tomographic (CT) or magnetic resonance (MR) angiography with contrast helps to assess arterial wall thickening as well as delineate anatomical stenotic (or rarely aneurysmal) arterial lesions. MR angiography without contrast (useful in individuals with renal failure) can help assess the anatomy of the arterial tree. Positron emission tomography (PET) using 18-F fluorodeoxyglucose (FDG) helps to assess metabolic activity in the aorta and its branches which indicate inflammatory activity of TAK. PET is usually combined with CT or MR for anatomical localization.

Treatment

Active disease in TAK is treated with immunosuppressive therapy. Identifying active disease in TAK is challenging and relies on a composite assessment of clinical features (constitutional features, carotidynia, new onset of pulse loss or vascular bruits), raised erythrocyte sedimentation rate (ESR) and/or C-reactive protein (CRP), and arterial FDG uptake on PET. However, these features individually do not well distinguish active or inactive TAK. Corticosteroids are the first-line immunosuppressive therapy, usually at a dose of 0.5 mg/kg/day, tapered over 6 months to 1 year to a dose of 5 mg daily or lesser, and stopped if possible. Along with corticosteroids, disease-modifying anti-rheumatic drugs (DMARDs), whether conventional, biologic, or targeted synthetic, are initiated (Table 41.1).

Table 41.1: Immunosuppressive therapies used for TAK		
Drug Name	*Dose*	*Toxicity/ Contraindications*
Corticosteroids	0.5 mg/kg/day	Cushingoid features, weight gain, diabetes mellitus
Methotrexate	Up to 25 mg/week	Cytopenias, transaminitis
Azathioprine	2 mg/kg/day	Cytopenias, transaminitis
Mycophenolate mofetil	2–3 gram/day	Cytopenias, transaminitis
Leflunomide	20 mg/day	Cytopenias, transaminitis
Tacrolimus	1–6 mg/day (titrated as per trough level)	Renal failure, hyperkalemia, diabetes mellitus, dyslipidemia
Cyclophosphamide	750 mg/m^2 monthly for 6 months	Cytopenias
TNF inhibitors	Infliximab 5 mg/kg 4 weekly, Adalimumab 40 mg fortnightly, 25 mg subcutaneous twice a week	Serious infections (including reactivation of tuberculosis), transaminitis
Tocilizumab	8 mg/kg intravenous monthly or 162 mg subcutaneous weekly	Transaminitis, serious infections, dyslipidemia, neutropenia
Tofacitinib	10 mg/day	Transaminitis
Baricitinib	4 mg/day	Transaminitis

Hypertension is a common feature of TAK, particularly in Asians, and is treated as usual. A point to note is the need to avoid angiotensin-converting enzyme inhibitors (ACEi) or angiotensin receptor blockers (ARBs) should be avoided when there is anatomical bilateral renal artery stenosis or even if the descending thoracic aorta or suprarenal abdominal aorta are involved without renal artery stenosis (functional bilateral renal artery stenosis). Antiplatelet agents are used for severe ischemic complications such as stroke, myocardial infarction, or ocular ischemia, or after endovascular procedures.

Due to extensive collateral vessel formation, most patients with TAK do not require revascularization procedures. Revascularization is only indicated for critical end-organ ischemia such as ischemic stroke, myocardial infarction, ischemic optic neuropathy, or acute abdominal angina, or with chronic ischemia affecting quality of life such as limb claudication, refractory renovascular hypertension or gradual decline in renal function with renal artery stenosis, or chronic abdominal angina. Balloon angioplasty is preferable to stenting for the renal arteries, stenting is better than angioplasty for coronary artery involvement in TAK, whereas, for the other arterial territories, either modality may be used. Aortic regurgitation or aneurysms at a risk of rupture might require endovascular or open surgical repair. Interventions should always be carried out in patients with TAK during periods of inactive disease for fear of complications such as restenosis or arterial wall rupture. Any patient with TAK undergoing endovascular intervention should be treated with antiplatelet agents unless there is a contraindication for these drugs.

Prognosis

TAK is associated with a markedly increased risk of dying when compared with the general population, based on data from India, Europe, and North American cohorts. Recent literature from India revealed a 5-year survival of 94% and a 10-year survival of 89%. Cardiovascular disease is the major cause of death in patients with TAK followed by infections. Pediatric-onset TAK (18 years) is associated with higher mortality risk.

Pregnancy is an important consideration in patients with TAK since this disease commonly affects young females. TAK is associated with an increased risk of fetal and maternal complications, particularly when there is involvement of the abdominal aorta.

Clinical Snippet

A 25-year-old female presented with pain in the left upper limb, worse on activity, for the past three months. Examination revealed feeble left upper limb pulses, bilateral carotid and left subclavian bruits, and hypertension in the right upper limb. Her ESR (68 mm/hour) and CRP (32 mg/L) were elevated. CT angiography revealed wall thickening with narrowing in the arch of aorta, descending thoracic aorta, abdominal aorta, left subclavian, common carotids, and both renal arteries. She was initiated on daily prednisolone (30 mg) with mycophenolate mofetil.

FURTHER READING

1. Misra DP, Singh K, Rathore U, Kavadichanda CG, Ora M, Jain N, et al. Management of Takayasu arteritis. *Best Pract Res Clin Rheumatol* 2023;37:101826.

2. Quinn KA, Misra DP, Sharma A, Porter A, Mason J, Grayson PC. Takayasu's Arteritis. In: Stone JH, ed. *A Clinician's Pearls & Myths in Rheumatology*. Cham: Springer International Publishing; 2023:447–64.

3. Grayson PC, Ponte C, Suppiah R, Robson JC, Gribbons KB, Judge A, et al. 2022 American College of Rheumatology/EULAR classification criteria for Takayasu arteritis. *Ann Rheum Dis* 2022;81:1654–1660.

4. Hellmich B, Agueda A, Monti S, Buttgereit F, de Boysson H, Brouwer E, et al. 2018 Update of the EULAR recommendations for the management of large vessel vasculitis. *Ann Rheum Dis*. 2020;79:19–30.

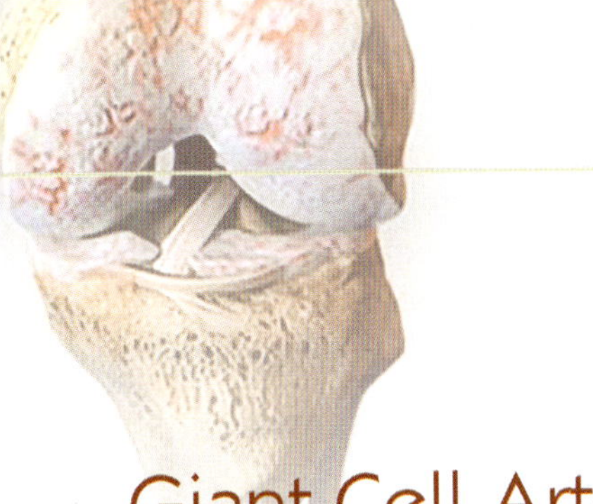

Giant Cell Arteritis

Phani Kumar D

INTRODUCTION

Giant cell arteritis (GCA), also known as temporal arteritis, is a systemic vasculitis predominantly affecting medium and large-sized arteries. It is most common in individuals aged over 50, particularly in women. The hallmark of GCA is inflammation of the temporal arteries, but it can involve large vessels. Early diagnosis and treatment are critical to prevent severe complications.

Clinical Features

The presentation of GCA is highly variable, making diagnosis challenging. The most common symptom is a new-onset headache, typically localised to the temporal region but may also be diffuse or occipital. The headache is often persistent and does not respond well to analgesics. Other cranial symptoms include scalp tenderness and jaw claudication due to ischemia of the masticatory muscles. Jaw claudication is highly suggestive of GCA.

Visual symptoms are among the most serious manifestations of GCA. Approximately 15–20% of patients experience partial or complete vision loss in one or both eyes, often due to anterior ischemic optic neuropathy (AION) caused by occlusion of the posterior ciliary artery. Transient visual loss, or amaurosis fugax, is also a concerning symptom that can progress to permanent blindness if not promptly treated with high-dose glucocorticoids.

In addition to cranial and visual symptoms, GCA may present with systemic manifestations such as fever, malaise, anorexia, and weight loss. These symptoms may be the sole indicators of the disease. Approximately 16% of patients with fever of unknown origin in individuals aged 65 and above are eventually diagnosed with GCA.

Diagnosis of Giant Cell Arteritis

The diagnosis of giant cell arteritis (GCA) is often complex due to its diverse clinical manifestations and potential for atypical presentations. Early diagnosis is crucial to prevent severe complications like irreversible vision loss.

Laboratory Testing

Key laboratory tests include elevated erythrocyte sedimentation rate (ESR) and C-reactive protein (CRP), which are hallmark findings in GCA. However, 5% of patients may have normal ESR levels. CRP is a more sensitive marker and should be used especially when ESR is normal. Other markers may include elevated fibrinogen, haptoglobin, and mild anemia. Autoimmune markers such as ANA, RF, and ANCAs are typically negative, helping to differentiate GCA from other conditions.

Temporal Artery Biopsy (TAB)

TAB remains the gold standard for diagnosing GCA, revealing granulomatous inflammation, intimal hyperplasia, and elastic lamina disruption. However, TAB has a sensitivity of around 85%, meaning a negative result does not exclude GCA. This is due to the "skip lesion" phenomenon, where unaffected areas may exist between inflamed segments.

Imaging Studies

When TAB is negative or not feasible, imaging studies are invaluable. Ultrasonography can detect the "halo sign," a specific indicator of GCA, particularly when bilateral. MRI and MRA are useful for evaluating large vessel involvement and detecting arterial wall edema. CTA is effective for assessing deep vessels like the aorta, though it involves radiation exposure. PET-CT, which detects increased FDG uptake, is highly sensitive and specific for large-vessel vasculitis but less effective for smaller arteries.

Classification Criteria

The American College of Rheumatology (ACR) /EULAR 2022 criteria for GCA assign points as follows: +5 for a positive temporal artery biopsy or halo sign on ultrasound; +3 for ESR 50 mm/hour, CRP 10 mg/litre, or sudden visual loss; and +2 for morning stiffness, jaw/tongue claudication, new temporal headache, scalp tenderness, abnormal temporal artery exam, bilateral axillary involvement on imaging, or FDG-PET activity in the aorta. A cumulative score of 6 or more points classifies a patient as having GCA.

Differential Diagnosis

Differential diagnoses include Takayasu arteritis, SLE, rheumatoid arthritis, and atherosclerosis. Accurate diagnosis requires ruling out these conditions through a comprehensive clinical and laboratory evaluation.

Treatment

The primary goal in treating giant cell arteritis (GCA) is to rapidly control inflammation and prevent complications, especially vision loss. High-dose glucocorticoids are the mainstay of therapy. Prednisone is typically started at 40–60 mg/day, with intravenous methylprednisolone (1000 mg daily for 3 days) reserved for acute visual loss. Once symptoms and inflammatory markers normalise, glucocorticoids are tapered gradually. The tapering process typically begins after 2–4 weeks, with careful monitoring for relapses.

For patients who experience relapses or significant side effects from glucocorticoids, immunosuppressive agents like methotrexate (7.5–15 mg weekly) and tocilizumab (162 mg/week SC) are used as steroid-sparing options. Methotrexate reduces the cumulative glucocorticoid dose, while tocilizumab is particularly beneficial in refractory cases.

Drug Name	Dose	Toxicity/Contraindication	Special Notes
Prednisone	40–60 mg/day	Hyperglycemia, hypertension, osteoporosis	Gradual tapering required
Methotrexate	7.5–25 mg/week	Hepatotoxicity, bone marrow suppression	Steroid-sparing agent, effective after 24 weeks
Tocilizumab	162 mg/week SC	Increased risk of infections, GI perforations	Consider in refractory cases or GC intolerance
Aspirin	75–150 mg/day	Increased bleeding risk	Role in preventing cranial ischemic complications is controversial

Adjunctive therapies include low-dose aspirin (75–150 mg/day) for preventing ischemic complications, though its use is debated. Patients on long-term glucocorticoids should receive calcium (1000–1500 mg/day) and vitamin D (800 IU/day) to prevent osteoporosis, with bisphosphonates recommended for those at high risk.

Prognosis

The prognosis of GCA varies, with most patients achieving remission with appropriate treatment. However, relapses are common, and some patients may require long-term low-dose corticosteroids. The disease does not generally affect overall survival except in cases with aortic involvement, which carries a risk of aortic dissection and aneurysm rupture. Early initiation of treatment is crucial in preventing complications, particularly visual loss, which is often irreversible once it occurs.

Clinical Snippet

A 72-year-old woman presented with a two-month history of new-onset headaches localised to the temporal region, associated with jaw claudication and transient visual loss in the left eye. Laboratory investigations revealed elevated ESR and CRP. Temporal artery biopsy confirmed GCA. She was initiated on 60 mg/day of prednisone, resulting in a rapid resolution of symptoms. Over the following months, the dose was gradually tapered, and she remained in remission at her six-month follow-up.

FURTHER READING

1. Ciofalo A, Gulotta G, Iannella G, Pasquariello B, Manno A, Angeletti D, Pace A, Greco A, Altissimi G, de Vincentiis M, Magliulo G. Giant Cell Arteritis (GCA): Pathogenesis, Clinical Aspects and Treatment Approaches. Curr Rheumatol Rev. 2019;15(4):259–68.
2. Galli E, Muratore F, Warrington KJ. Current management of giant cell arteritis and its complications. Curr Opin Rheumatol. 2024 Sep 1;36(5):344–50.

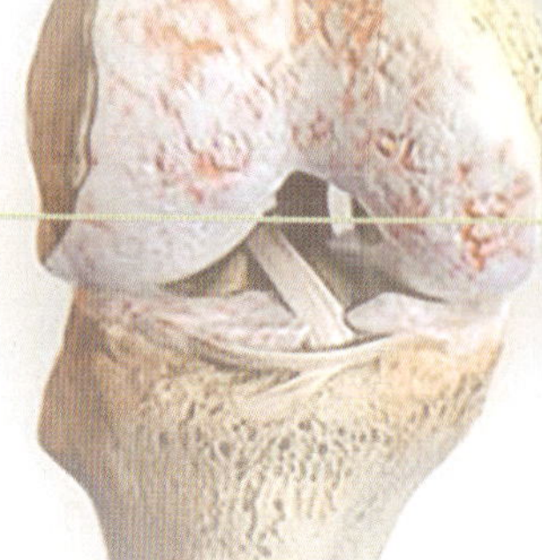

Polyarteritis Nodosa

VN Nagaprabhu, Vellamal P

INTRODUCTION

Polyarteritis nodosa (PAN) is a form of necrotizing vasculitis predominantly affecting medium size vessels with heterogeneous manifestations. Historically, PAN was linked to HBV hepatitis B virus infection, but this has changed recently due to declining HBV prevalence and now there is a connection between PAN and genetic syndromes as well as malignancies.

With the better understanding of the underlying pathogenesis PAN is now known to have various subtypes:

1. Classical PAN
2. Cutaneous PAN
3. PAN associated with HBV or other infections
4. PAN with DADA2 mutations
5. PAN associated with malignancies/myelodysplastic syndrome

Clinical Features

Clinical features of PAN results from damage to vascular walls affecting all organs. The commonest presenting feature is general, non-specific symptoms such as fever, weight loss, and arthralgia. The next most common system is neurological seen in around two-third of the patients, presenting as the characteristic motor and sensory mononeuritis multiplexa or as polyneuropathy. Cranial nerves are less commonly involved and central nervous system manifestations are rare except those associated with DADA2.

Cutaneous skin lesions like purpura, nodules, necrotic ulcers and livedo reticularis are seen in half of the patients. Renal involvement characterized by stenosis and aneurysms primarily affecting the renal and interlobular arteries, which presents as hypertension, micro- or macrohematuria and renal infarct. Glomerular involvement is not seen. Gastrointestinal manifestations can be seen in up to 50% of patients with vascular inflammation in the mesenteric arteries. Testicular pain with or without orchitis is specific to PAN. Cardiovascular involvement is seen due to coronary artery vasculitis.

Diagnosis

The diagnosis of PAN is based on the classification criteria proposed by American College of Rheumatology 1999 classification and also 2012 revised classification criteria by Chapel Hill consensus (CHC) nomenclature.

CHC definition: Necrotizing arteritis of medium or small arteries without glomerulo-nephritis or vasculitis in arterioles, capillaries or venules and not associated with ANCA positivity.

ACR 1999 Criteria

3 out of 10

1. Weight loss above 4 kg
2. Diastolic blood pressure above 99 mm Hg
3. HBV positivity
4. Mononeuropathy/polyneuropathy
5. Elevated urea creatinine
6. Testicular pain/tenderness
7. Livedo reticularis
8. Myalgias
9. Arteriographic abnormality
10. Biopsy of a small or medium-sized artery containing polymorphonuclear neutrophils.

Treatment

The treatment of PAN depends upon association with underlying HBV-hepatitis B virus infection, which is nowadays becoming rare. The management of PAN without systemic involvement and FFS score of 0 is usually with low dose steroids and immunosuppressants are indicated only for steroid sparing effect or for those with severe disease.

Systemic Involvement (FFS score >0) PAN without HBV infection

Drug	Dose	Toxicity	Contraindication	Special Notes
Corticosteroids (high dose)	1 mg/kg	Metabolic effects (change in blood sugars, calcium etc.) elevated blood pressures, increased infection risk	Uncontrolled blood sugars, active infection	First line drug for induction
Cyclophosphamide	500 mg (1, 15 & 29 days-every 3 weeks)	Cytopenia, gonadal toxicity, infection risk	Active infection, planning pregnancy	Reserved for induction in severe cases
Azathioprine	2–3 mg/kg per day	Cytopenia, infection risk	Active infection	Maintenance therapy
Methotrexate	0.3 mg/kg per week	Cytopenia, infection risk, gonadal toxicity	Active infection	Steroid sparing
Plasma exchange	60 ml/kg 3–4 times per week (for 3 weeks)			Cases refractory to standard therapies

Prognosis

The 1996 version of the five factor score (FFS) can be used for risk stratification in this proteinuria greater than 1 gm/day, Sr.Creatinine more than 1.58 mg/dl, cardiomyopathy, severe gastrointestinal involvement and CNS involvement are scored with one point each.FFS score of 0 is considered as mild PAN and anything more than 1 has higher risk of mortality.

FURTHER READING

1. Wolff L, Horisberger A, Moi L, Karampetsou MP, Comte D. Polyarteritis Nodosa: Old Disease, New Etiologies. Int J Mol Sci. 2023 Nov 23;24(23):16668. doi: 10.3390/ijms242316668. PMID: 38068989; PMCID: PMC10706353.

2. Terrier B, Darbon R, Durel CA, Hachulla E, Karras A, Maillard H, Papo T, Puechal X, Pugnet G, Quemeneur T, Samson M, Taille C, Guillevin L; Collaborators. French recommendations for the management of systemic necrotizing vasculitides (polyarteritis nodosa and ANCA-associated vasculitides). Orphanet J Rare Dis. 2020 Dec 29;15(Suppl 2):351. doi: 10.1186/s13023-020-01621-3.

3. Karadag O, Jayne DJ. Polyarteritis nodosa revisited: a review of historical approaches, subphenotypes and a research agenda. Clin Exp Rheumatol. 2018 Mar-Apr;36 Suppl 111(2):135-142. Epub 2018 Feb 20. PMID: 29465365.

Granulomatosis with Polyangiitis

Keerthi Talari Bommakanti, Pravin Hissaria

INTRODUCTION

Granulomatosis with polyangiitis (GPA), previously called Wegener's granulomatosis, is a form of small- to medium-vessel vasculitis. This autoimmune disease is marked by necrotizing inflammation and granuloma formation, primarily affecting the respiratory tract and kidneys, though it may involve multiple organ systems. Classified within the anti-neutrophil cytoplasmic antibody (ANCA)-associated vasculitides (AAV), GPA is characterized by PR3-ANCA or c-ANCA positivity in most patients. The exact etiology remains unknown, though a combination of genetic predisposition and environmental factors likely contributes to its onset.

Clinical Features

The clinical manifestations of GPA are diverse, reflecting the variable organ involvement typical of vasculitis. Early symptoms often involve the respiratory tract, but systemic and renal features become more prominent as the disease progresses.

- **Upper respiratory tract:** Common symptoms include chronic rhinosinusitis, nasal crusting, and recurrent epistaxis (nosebleeds). Nasal septal perforation and saddle-nose deformity, resulting from cartilage destruction, are distinctive features that may develop in untreated or chronic cases.
- **Lower respiratory tract:** Pulmonary involvement in GPA presents as persistent cough, hemoptysis (coughing up blood), and pleuritic chest pain. Imaging studies frequently reveal nodules, infiltrates, or cavitary lesions. Pulmonary hemorrhage, although rare, can be life-threatening. Lung biopsies often demonstrate necrotizing granulomatous inflammation.
- **Renal involvement:** Approximately 80% of GPA patients develop kidney involvement over time, typically in the form of rapidly progressive glomerulonephritis. This manifests as hematuria, proteinuria, and progressive renal insufficiency, which can lead to renal failure if untreated. Renal biopsy often reveals pauci-immune crescentic glomerulonephritis.
- **Constitutional Features:** Fever, weight loss, fatigue and loss of appetite.
- **Other organ involvement:**
  - *Eyes:* Inflammation can affect the eyes, resulting in scleritis, episcleritis, or, orbital pseudotumor. These can lead to vision disturbances and are often painful.

- *Skin:* Cutaneous involvement may present as purpura, nodules, and ulcers due to small-vessel vasculitis.
- *Nervous system:* Peripheral neuropathy or mononeuritis multiplex can occur due to nerve ischemia.
- *Musculoskeletal system:* Arthralgia and arthritis are frequently reported, though they are typically non-erosive.

Classification Criteria

The 2022 ACR/EULAR classification criteria1 for GPA employ a points-based system, developed to improve the precision of GPA diagnosis in clinical research by differentiating it from other types of vasculitis. A cumulative score of 5 or more points classifies a patient as having GPA. The criteria are as follows:

1. **Bloody nasal discharge, nasal crusting, or sino-nasal congestion:** +3 points
2. **Cartilaginous involvement (e.g., saddle-nose deformity):** +2 points
3. **Conductive or sensorineural hearing loss:** +1 point
4. **Cytoplasmic ANCA (c-ANCA) or anti-proteinase 3 (PR3-ANCA) positivity:** +5 points
5. **Pulmonary nodules, masses, or cavitations on chest imaging:** +2 points
6. **Granuloma or giant cells on biopsy:** +2 points
7. **Nasal or paranasal sinus inflammation or consolidation on imaging:** +1 point
8. **Pauci-immune glomerulonephritis:** +1 point
9. **Perinuclear ANCA (p-ANCA) or anti-myeloperoxidase (MPO-ANCA) positivity:** -1 point
10. **Eosinophil count $\geq 1 \times 10^9$/L:** –4 points

Investigations

Diagnosis involves a combination of laboratory, imaging, and histopathological findings:

- **ANCA testing:** PR3-ANCA (c-ANCA) is present in 80–90% of GPA patients, and its presence is heavily weighted in the classification criteria. However, the absence of ANCA does not exclude GPA. It is usually tested in a two stage method with IIF and antigen specific ELISA tests. As a minimum, PR3 ELISA test is the most useful test to diagnose this condition.
- **Blood tests:** Elevated inflammatory markers, such as ESR and CRP, as well as normocytic anemia and leukocytosis, are common findings in active disease.
- **Urinalysis:** Kidney involvement may manifest as microscopic hematuria, proteinuria, or red blood cell casts in urinalysis, indicating glomerulonephritis.
- **Imaging:** Chest X-rays and CT scans are useful for identifying pulmonary nodules, cavitations, or infiltrates. Sinus imaging can reveal mucosal thickening, sinusitis, or other nasal changes.
- **Histopathology:** Tissue biopsy, often from the lung or kidney, should be done where feasible and can confirm granulomatous inflammation and necrotizing vasculitis.

Treatment

Management of GPA consists of induction and maintenance therapy phases, aimed at achieving and sustaining remission.

GPA is classified based on the extent of organ involvement and disease severity:
- **Localized:** Limited to the upper and/or lower respiratory tract.
- **Early systemic:** Involvement of non-life-threatening organs, without major renal involvement.
- **Generalized:** More extensive disease, typically involving kidneys.
- **Severe:** Life-threatening, with critical organ dysfunction.
- **Refractory:** Disease that persists or recurs despite appropriate treatment.

Induction Therapy

The goal of induction therapy is to suppress active inflammation quickly to prevent irreversible organ damage:
- **Glucocorticoids:** High-dose glucocorticoids, such as prednisone, are used initially, often with a rapid taper based on the patient's response.
- **Cyclophosphamide or rituximab:** For severe GPA, cyclophosphamide or rituximab is administered alongside glucocorticoids. Both drugs are effective in achieving remission, with rituximab offering a favorable side-effect profile, particularly for relapsing cases. Cyclophosphamide is usually reserved for more severe renal disease.
- **Plasma exchange (plasmapheresis):** For patients with severe renal involvement or life-threatening pulmonary hemorrhage, plasma exchange may be beneficial. It helps remove ANCA antibodies and other inflammatory mediators.
- **Methotrexate:** May be considered for localised disease
- Avacopan, a C5AR antagonist, is a recent addition to the treatment algorithm in the induction therapy of AAV. It has been shown to have a steroid sparing effect and is particularly useful when high dose steroids are relatively contraindicated.

Maintenance Therapy

After remission, maintenance therapy helps reduce the risk of relapse:
- **Azathioprine, methotrexate, or rituximab:** These agents are commonly used for long-term maintenance. Azathioprine and methotrexate are options for patients without severe renal impairment, while rituximab is often preferred for patients with high relapse risk.

  Preventative measures, like Pneumocystis pneumonia prophylaxis during high-dose immunosuppression, are essential.

Prognosis

The prognosis of GPA has significantly improved with advances in immunosuppressive therapy, with many patients achieving remission. However, relapses are common, especially among PR3-ANCA-positive patients or those with lung involvement. Long-term follow-up is essential, with attention to relapse, treatment-related complications, and chronic organ damage, particularly in the kidneys.

Clinical Snippet

A 55-year-old patient presents with chronic sinusitis, recurrent nasal crusting, persistent cough with hemoptysis, and unexplained hematuria. Imaging reveals pulmonary nodules, and laboratory tests show elevated PR3-ANCA. Lung biopsy confirms granulomatous inflammation. With a cumulative score meeting the 2022 classification criteria for GPA, the patient is diagnosed and started on induction therapy with glucocorticoids and rituximab, highlighting the importance of prompt and targeted treatment in GPA management.

FURTHER READING

1. Robson JC, Grayson PC, Ponte C, Suppiah R, Craven A, Judge A, et al. 2022 American College of Rheumatology/European Alliance of Associations for Rheumatology classification criteria for granulomatosis with polyangiitis. Ann Rheum Dis. 2022;81:315–320. doi: 10.1136/annrheumdis-2021-221795

2. Hellmich B, Sanchez-Alamo B, Schirmer JH, Berti A, Blockmans D, Cid MC, Holle JU, Hollinger N, Karadag O, Kronbichler A, Little MA, Luqmani RA, Mahr A, Merkel PA, Mohammad AJ, Monti S, Mukhtyar CB, Musial J, Price-Kuehne F, Segelmark M, Teng YKO, Terrier B, Tomasson G, Vaglio A, Vassilopoulos D, Verhoeven P, Jayne D. EULAR recommendations for the management of ANCA-associated vasculitis: 2022 update. Ann Rheum Dis. 2024 Jan 2;83(1):30-47. doi: 10.1136/ard-2022-223764. PMID:36927642.

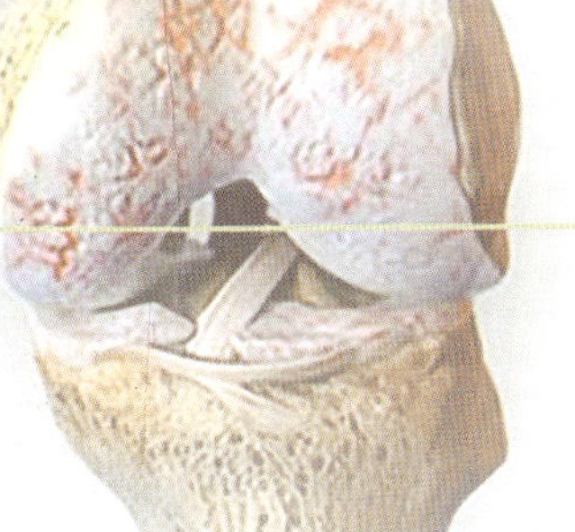

Eosinophilic Granulomatosis with Polyangiitis

Amirtha Gopalan

INTRODUCTION

Eosinophilic granulomatosis with polyangiitis (EGPA), formerly Churg-Strauss syndrome is the rarest form of ANCA-associated vasculitis. It is characterised by late-onset asthma, peripheral and tissue eosinophilia, extravascular granuloma formation, and vasculitis of multiple organ systems.

Clinical Features

EGPA is equally prevalent in men and women and the mean age at diagnosis is around 50 years. EGPA typically (but not necessarily) occurs in 3 phases:

1. **Prodromal:** Usually in the 3rd decade of life. Late-onset asthma, allergic rhinitis, sinusitis, peripheral eosinophilia >1500/mm³, migratory arthralgia, and myalgia are typical.
2. **Eosinophilic:** There is increasing eosinophilia and eosinophilic tissue infiltration of organs (lungs and intestines).
3. **Vasculitic:** Systemic vasculitis typically affecting the skin, nerves and kidneys.

   These three phases do not necessarily follow one another in this order. The average length of time between diagnosis of asthma and vasculitis is 4 to 9 years.

Organ Involvement in EGPA

General symptoms, such as fever, weight loss, arthralgia and malaise are present in most patients.

Organ	Manifestations	Incidence
Upper respiratory tract	Rhinitis, sinusitis, nasal polyposis	75%
	Destructive lesions rarely occur	
Lower respiratory tract	Asthma-late onset, can be severe and refractory to treatment	90%
	Patchy and fleeting pulmonary infiltrates (non-cavitating)	75%
	Eosinophilic pleural effusions	
	Diffuse alveolar hemorrhage (in ANCA+)	10%
Neurological system	Mononeuritis multiplex	75%
	Distal symmetric sensorimotor polyneuropathy	20%
	CNS involvement is uncommon	

(Contd.)

(Contd.)

Organ	Manifestations	Incidence
Cardiovascular system	Myocarditis Pericarditis Heart failure Arrhythmias	15–20%
Gastrointestinal system	Eosinophilic gastroenteritis-bleeding pain abdomen Cholecystitis	20–30%
Skin	Palpable purpura Nodules Livedo Churg-Strauss granuloma	30%

ANCA positive EGPA patents are more likely to have vasculitic features like glomerulonephritis, alveolar hemorrhage and peripheral nerve involvement. ANCA negative patients with EGPA are more prone to cardiac involvement and experience higher mortality.

Diagnosis

There is no single diagnostic test of choice for EGPA. Peripheral blood eosinophilia (greater than 10% on differential white blood cell count or greater than 1500/dl) is the best-known lab hallmark of the disease. Elevated serum IgE is also found in 75% of patients. ANCA is positive in 30–40% of patients and the common pattern is perinuclear.

Non-specific laboratory findings include anemia, leucocytosis, thrombocytosis, and elevated ESR or CRP. Abnormal urinary sediment may point towards glomerulonephritis. Airflow obstruction is present in pulmonary function tests in 70% of patients. Since cardiac disease portends a poor prognosis, screening with 2D-ECHO at the time of diagnosis is recommended.

Histopathological confirmation must be sought when feasible. Biopsy of skin, sural nerve, kidney, lung aid in diagnosis. The hallmarks of histopathological findings in EGPA are

1. **Vasculitis:** Fibrinoid necrosis and rupture of the internal elastic lamina in small and medium-sized vessels.
2. Eosinophilic infiltrates.
3. Perivascular and extravascular granulomas.

However, these histological findings are not always found together or at the same site.

Management of EGPA

The vasculitis and asthma manifestations of EGPA are usually managed distinctly. Asthma treatment generally follows conventional asthma management guidelines including avoidance of allergens, inhaled therapies and antihistamines. Treatment of vasculitis is typically based on a patient's disease features and severity and includes glucocorticoids with immunosuppressives. Collaboration between rheumatologists and asthma/allergy specialists can enhance the care of patients with EGPA.

Treatment of Vasculitic Manifestations

A frequently used system to assess the severity and prognosis of vasculitis is the revised five-factor score (FFS) which includes:

- Age >65 years,
- Elevation of serum creatinine (>1.70 mg/dl),
- Symptomatic cardiac insufficiency,
- Severe gastrointestinal manifestations
- The absence of ENT involvement.

FFS >1 is considered to be a severe disease, with a one-year survival rate of 60%. The clinical profile of nonsevere EGPA includes predominantly asthma, sinus disease, and nonsevere vasculitis.

Severity of disease	Induction	Maintenance
Active severe disease	IV pulse methylprednisolone Cyclophosphamide or Rituximab	Methotrexate or Azathioprine or Mycophenolate mofetyl
Active non-severe disease	GC + Mepolizumab* or GC + Methotrexate or GC + Azathioprine or GC + Mycophenolate mofetyl or GC + Rituximab	Methotrexate or Azathioprine or Mycophenolate mofetyl
Relapse	Consider a different immunosuppressive based on clinical features and patient factors	

*Mepolizumab is an anti-IL-5 monoclonal antibody which can be used for maintenance therapy in patients with asthma and sinonasal disease.

The duration of glucocorticoid or immunosuppressive therapy is not clear and should be guided by patient clinical features.

Clinical Vignette

A 42-year-old male presented with a history of shortness of breath for 6 months. It was associated with orthopnea and swelling of both lower limbs. He also gave a history of tingling numbness in his right leg and foot for 3 months followed by a right foot drop 1 week back. He had asthma since the age of 23 years and recurrent sinus infections for which he used multiple inhalers, antihistamines and oral steroids. On examination, he had pitting pedal edema, elevated JVP, fine crepitations in both lung fields, and right foot drop with reduced sensation in the right foot and leg.

The patient's reports revealed raised inflammatory markers, eosinophilia (count of 1600/mm^3), raised serum IgE level, normal renal and liver function tests, CT chest showed 2 small non-cavitating pulmonary nodules and a mild pleural effusion, 2D ECHO showed LV global hypokinesia with EF of 17%. ANCA was negative. Sural nerve biopsy showed marked perivascular inflammation with lymphocytes and eosinophils suggestive of vasculitis.

A diagnosis of EGPA (ANCA negative) with myocarditis, mononeuritis multiplex, lung involvement was made. He was treated with glucocorticoids and monthly cyclophosphamide pulses for 6 months and is currently in remission with maintenance on azathioprine.

Prognosis

Following timely detection and treatment, EGPA has a favourable prognosis with a 5-year survival rate reaching 90%. Asthma often remains refractory and impacts the quality of life. Management of patients with severe vasculitis, cardiomyopathy, and renal failure at presentation remains a challenge. Infection is a major problem, especially in the early course of disease. Relapses occur in 20 to 30% of patients, risk factors for relapse include sudden rise in eosinophil count, persistent ANCA positivity or rise in titres, and gastrointestinal tract (GI) involvement.

FURTHER READING

1. White J, Dubey S. Eosinophilic granulomatosis with polyangiitis: A review. Autoimmun Rev. 2023 Jan;22(1):103219.
2. Hellmich B, Sanchez-Alamo B, Schirmer JH, et al. EULAR recommendations for the management of ANCA-associated vasculitis: 2022 update Annals *of the Rheumatic Diseases* 2024;83:30–47.

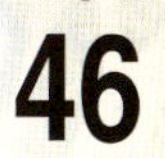

Microscopic Polyangiitis

Madhuri HR

INTRODUCTION

Microscopic polyangiitis (MPA) is a necrotizing small vessel vasculitis, classified under antineutrophil cytoplasmic antibodies (ANCA) vasculitis along with granulomatous polyangiitis (GPA) and eosinophilic granulomatosis with polyangiitis (EGPA). Previously, the terms polyarteritis nodosa, microscopic polyarteritis, and microscopic polyangiitis were considered the same. In 1948, the term microscopic polyangiitis was introduced by Davson to describe glomerulonephritis in patients with polyarteritis nodosa.

Clinical Features

There is a slight male predominance with an average age of onset of 50–60 years. Constitutional features like fever, weight loss, and arthralgias are very common. Clinical features are summarised in Table 46.1.

Table 46.1: Clinical features of microscopic polyangiitis			
Organ	Incidence	Common manifestations	Life-threatening manifestations
Renal	80%	Proteinuria, hematuria	Rapidly progressive glomerulonephritis
Pulmonary	10%	Alveolar hemorrhage, pulmonary fibrosis	Catastrophic pulmonary hemorrhage (10%)
Skin	30–60%	Palpable purpura, nodules, ulcers, digital gangrene	
Gastrointestinal	30–58%	Pain abdomen, colonic ulcers, intestinal ischemia	bowel perforation, gastrointestinal bleed
Neurological	37–72%	Peripheral neuropathy, mononeuritis multiplex, cranial neuropathy, cerebral hemorrhage, pachymeningitis, cerebral infarcts	
Rare		Scleritis, episcleritis, pericarditis, myocardial infarction	Congestive cardiac failure

Diagnosis

ANCA antibodies to MPO are present in the majority of the cases. ELISA is now the preferred method for ANCA testing. Anti-MPO antibodies are found in 70–90% and anti-PR3 antibodies may be found in around 20% of MPA cases.

Definitive diagnosis is by histopathology, renal biopsy, skin and sural nerve are the easily accessible sites with good yield. Kidney biopsy shows pauci-immune crescentic, focal segmental glomerulonephritis. The small-medium vessels may show fibrinoid necrosis in other tissues. Granulomas are not seen.

Routine investigations suggest an inflammatory process with anemia, leucocytosis and thrombocytosis on the hemogram and elevated ESR and CRP. Microscopic urine abnormalities are seen in the majority, hematuria, proteinuria and red cell casts may be seen.

Chest imaging by CT scan may be needed in suspicious pulmonary involvement.

The ACR/EULAR 2022 classification criteria is given in Table 46.2. A sum of 5 or more is needed to classify as MPA.

Table 46.2: ACR/EUCAR 2022 classification criteria	
Criteria	*Points*
Nasal involvement, including bloody discharge, ulcers, crusting, congestion, blockage, or septal defect/perforation	–3
Positive test for p-ANCA or anti-MPO ANCA	+6
Fibrosis or interstitial lung disease on chest imaging	+3
Pauci-immune glomerulonephritis on biopsy	+3
Positive test for c-ANCA or anti-PR3 ANCA	–1
Blood eosinophil count $\geq 1 \times 10^9$/L	–4

Treatment

The EULAR 2022 recommendations for management of MPA are given below.

Induction phase for organ or life-threatening disease is by glucocorticoids and either rituximab or cyclophosphamide. In non-organ-threatening or non-life-threatening diseases and new-onset diseases, mycophenolate mofetil or methotrexate can be considered with glucocorticoids. Rituximab is preferred in relapsing disease.

Glucocorticoids are given at oral doses of 50–75 mg/day prednisolone equivalent and tapered to achieve a dose of 5 mg per day by 4–5 months. PLEX may be considered to induce remission in acute renal failure or diffuse alveolar hemorrhage, though the evidence is not conclusive.

Maintenance of remission is usually with rituximab or azathioprine. Mycophenolate mofetil or methotrexate may be used in selected cases. The EULAR guidelines recommend therapy to maintain remission for MPA be continued for 24–48 months following induction of remission of new-onset disease. Longer duration of therapy should be considered in relapsing patients or those with an increased risk of relapse, but should be balanced against patient preferences and risks of continuing immunosuppression.

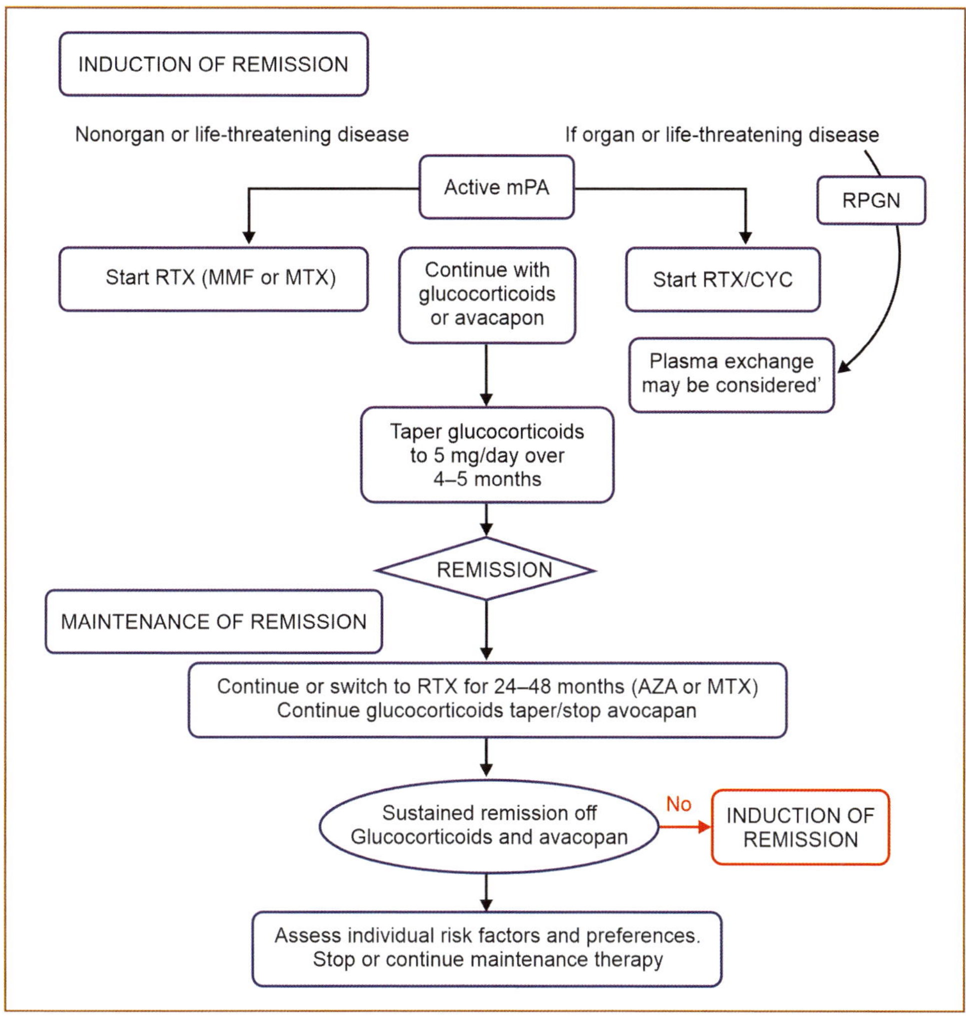

Fig 46.1: Outline of management of microscopic polyangiitis. MTX: Methotrexate; RTX: Rituximab; CYC: Cyclophosphamide; AZA: Azathioprine; MMF: Mycophenolate mofetyl

Toxicity Concerns

Drug	Toxicity concerns
Glucocorticoids	Weight gain, diabetes, osteoporosis, GI bleeds
Cyclophosphamide	Decrease in ovarian reserve, cytopenias, infection, caution in women of reproductive age group
Azathioprine	Bone marrow suppression, hepatotoxicity, infection
Mycophenolate Mofetil	Needs monitoring of cell counts and liver function tests, infection, caution in women of reproductive age group
Methotrexate	Cytopenias, hepatotoxicity, alopecia, caution in women of reproductive age group
Rituximab	Hypogammaglobulinemia, blunted vaccine responses, infection

Prognosis

One-year survival rates are 82–92% and five-year survival rates range between 45–76%. Renal involvement confers a higher risk of mortality. The mortality is higher in the initial few months of illness. Relapses are common in MPA. Comorbidities like cardiovascular events, cerebrovascular accidents and thromboembolic events are higher as the duration increases.

Clinical Snippet

A 60-year-old female presented with mild hemoptysis and breathlessness for 2 days. She had a history of on-and-off fever, joint pains, and fatigue for 2 weeks and scattered red spots on the lower limbs for a month. Examination revealed a palpable purpuric rash on the legs and bilateral crepts on auscultation. Investigations showed leucocytosis (15,000/cu.mm), thrombocytosis and proteinuria. CT scan of the chest showed ground glass opacities.

ANA testing was negative and ANCA testing by IF showed a perinuclear pattern. Anti-MPO antibodies were elevated.

Management: This lady needs a renal biopsy or skin biopsy to confirm the diagnosis of MPA. Detailed neurological examination should be done and nerve conduction studies, if needed. Lung evaluation should be done to rule out infection (sputum and bronchoscopic lavage and biopsy if feasible). Treatment will be initiated with prednisolone at 1 mg/kg body weight and options of cyclophosphamide or rituximab are to be discussed. After induction and remission, maintenance with rituximab is recommended.

FURTHER READING

1. Hellmich B, Sanchez-Alamo B, Schirmer JH, et al. EULAR recommendations for the management of ANCA-associated vasculitis: 2022 update Annals of the Rheumatic Diseases 2024;83:30–47.
2. Chung SA, Langford CA, Maz M, et al. 2021 American College of Rheumatology/Vasculitis Foundation Guideline for the Management of Antineutrophil Cytoplasmic Antibody-Associated Vasculitis. Arthritis Rheumatol. 2021;73(8):1366–1383. doi:10.1002/art.41773.

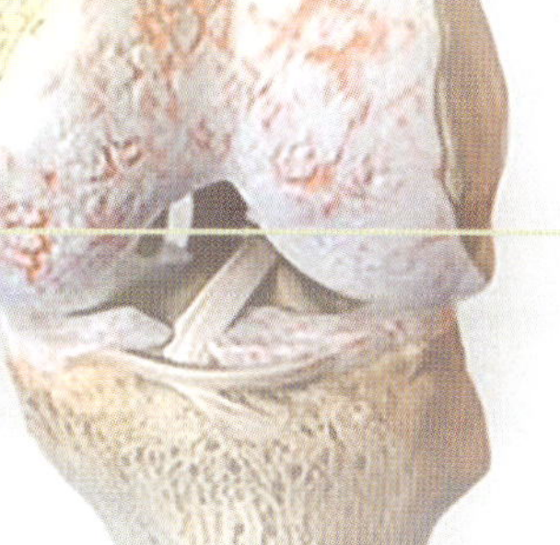

Kawasaki Disease

Sirisha K

INTRODUCTION

Kawasaki disease (mucocutaneous lymph node syndrome) is the most common medium vessel vasculitis affecting children below 5 years. Development of coronary artery abnormalities (15–25% of untreated cases) is responsible for the morbidity and mortality associated with the disease.

Epidemiology

The maximum incidence (264/100,000 children <5 years) of kawasaki disease (KD) is noticed in Japan. A hospital-based study in India showed varying incidence (1.0 in 2012, 9.1/100,000 in 2009). It is more common in children <5 years. Seasonal fluctuations in KD have been reported all over the world.

Etiopathogenesis

The underlying pathogenic mechanisms are unknown although a genetic basis, involvement of gut microbiota and infective agents have been proposed.

Clinical Features

The diagnosis of kawasaki disease is essentially clinical. Classic KD is diagnosed when fever lasts for more than 5 days in the presence of ≥4 principal clinical features (Table 47.1). Some clinical signs that are not included in diagnostic criteria but provide important clues to the diagnosis are listed in Table 47.2.

Incomplete Kawasaki Disease

Patients who do not meet sufficient diagnostic criteria for KD are said to have incomplete Kawasaki disease. It is more common in infants and older children. Treatment must be initiated promptly as delay in diagnosis may lead to adverse outcomes.

Natural Course

The natural course of kawasaki disease is often divided into the following 3 phases (Fig. 47.1).

Table 47.1: Principal clinical features of kawasaki disease (EULAR/PRES classification criteria for kawasaki disease).

Principal clinical feature	Remarks
Fever lasting for more than 5 days plus 4 of the following criteria	
1. Changes in peripheral extremities and perineal area	Erythema of hands and soles Painful induration and swelling of hands or feet Periungual desquamation
2. Bilateral subconjunctival injection	Bilateral, non-purulent, painless Spares the limbus
3. Polymorphous rash	Most common—diffuse macular papular eruption Other common forms—scarlatiniform erythroderma, erythema multiforme like Extensive rash involving trunk and extremities with early desquamation Uncommon—bullous, vesicular and petechial rash
4. Changes in oral mucosa	Lips—erythema, dryness, fissuring, peeling, cracking and bleeding Strawberry tongue Diffuse erythema of oropharyngeal mucosa Uncommon—oral ulcers, pharyngeal exudates
5. Cervical adenopathy	Unilateral, ≥1.5 cm in diameter Least common principal feature

Table 47.2: Fever lasting for more than 5 days plus 4 of the following criteria

Clinical sign	Note
1. Perineal desquamation	Occurs in the first week
2. Reactivation of the Bacillus Calmette–Guérin (BCG) injection site	Pathognomonic clinical sign
3. Extreme irritability	Noted especially in infants
4. Sterile pyuria Peripheral arthritis Hydrops of gallbladder Myocarditis	Other important indicators

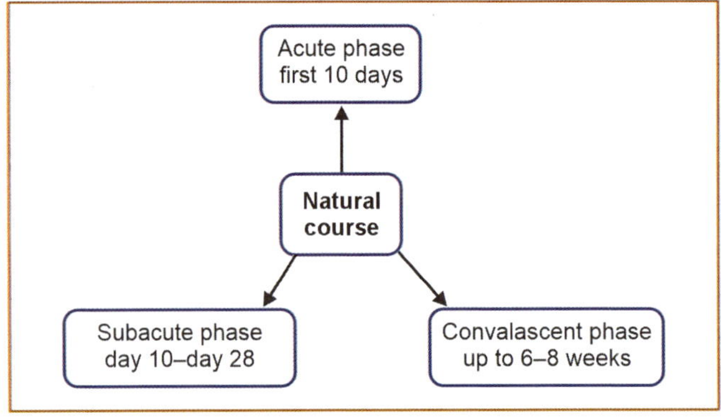

Fig 47.1: Types of natural course of Kawasaki disease

Investigations

There is no pathognomonic laboratory parameter. Laboratory investigations which aid in the diagnosis are as follows (*see* Table 47.3).

Differential Diagnosis

The differential diagnosis to KD is wide and include viral infections, drug hypersensitivity, juvenile idiopathic arthritis, staphylococcal scalded skin syndrome, Stevens-Johnson syndrome, streptococcal scarlet fever, toxic shock syndrome, etc.

However, the major hurdles in making a diagnosis of KD are:
1. Not considering the diagnosis upfront,
2. Seeking multiple consultations with different healthcare facilities (clinical signs might have disappeared or not documented).

Management

The ultimate goal of the therapy is to reduce coronary abnormalities given the availability of IVIG that can reduce the risk of coronary artery abnormalities from 23% to <5%. Table 47.4 covers the treatment options for Kawasaki disease.

Conclusion

It is the most common childhood acquired heart disease in developed countries. Sound knowledge of the clinical features is essential as the laboratory investigations are not pathognomonic. Time is the key as administration of IVIG along with aspirin will significantly prevent coronary abnormalities.

Table 47.3: Evaluation of kawasaki disease	
Laboratory investigations	*Remarks*
1. Comprehensive search for infective focus Blood culture Urinalysis and culture Chest x-ray Ultrasound abdomen	
2. **Inflammatory markers** ESR	Non specific As IVIG may increase ESR, it should not be used to assess response post treatment nonspecific
CRP Polymorphonuclear leukocytosis, normocytic anemia, thrombocytosis	Better marker to assess response post IVIG Acute phase reaction, consistently observed in 2nd or 3rd weeks
3. Echocardiography	Mandatory in acute phase to monitor cardiac complications (coronary artery dilatation and aneurysm, myocarditis) Normal study never rules out KD

Table 47.4: Management of kawasaki disease

Drug	Indication	Dosage	Duration	Remarks
IV Immunoglobulin	Persistent fever Signs of inflammation aneurysm on echocardiography	Single dose of 2 g/kg	Within 10 days of illness It is reasonable to administer beyond 10th day in case of persistent unexplained fever, coronary artery abnormalities with ongoing systemic inflammation.	Prevents the development of coronary aneurysms Second infusion in refractory KD
Aspirin		High dose of aspirin of 80 to 100 mg/day divided into 4 doses followed by low dose 3 to 5 mg/kg/day as a single dose	Until the patient is afebrile for 48 to 72 h. 6 to 8 weeks after the onset of the disease. Long term antiplatelet therapy for large aneurysms along with warfarin or low molecular weight heparin	Modifies the inflammatory status (at high doses) and prevents the risk of thrombosis (at low doses) Given along with IV IG Continued in case of persistent coronary abnormalities No definite evidence that aspirin can prevent coronary abnormalities.
Corticosteroids	High risk acute KD KD not responding to 2 or more infusions of IV IG	Prednisolone 2 mg/kg/day IV Pulse Methyl Prednisolone 20–30 mg/kg	8th hourly until afebrile followed by oral taper weeks Over 3 days with or without oral tapering over 2–3 weeks	Given together with IV IG and aspirin
TNF-α inhibitors	Refractory KD	Infliximab 5 mg/kg	Single dose	As an alternative to second infusion of IV IG or corticosteroids for refractory KD
Cyclosporin	Refractory KD	IV 3 mg/kg/day every 12 hours Oral 4-8 mg per kg per day every 12 hours	Tapered once afebrile, improving or CRP <1 mg/dl or after 2 weeks	KD refractory to second IV IG, infliximab or corticosteroids

Other alternative treatments: Anakinra, cyclophosphamide, plasma exchange
Refractory KD: Defined as persistent fever not responding to IVIG 36 hours after administration.

FURTHER READING

1. McCrindle BW et al. American Heart Association Rheumatic Fever, Endocarditis, and Kawasaki Disease Committee. Diagnosis, Treatment, and Long-Term Management of Kawasaki Disease: A Scientific Statement for Health Professionals From the American Heart Association. Circulation. 2017 Apr 25;135(17):e927-e999.
2. Ozen S, Ruperto N, Dillon MJ, et al. EULAR/PRES endorsed consensus criteria for the classification of childhood vasculitides. Ann Rheum Dis. 2006 Jul;65(7):936–41.
3. Singh S, Jindal AK, Pilania RK. Diagnosis of Kawasaki disease. Int J Rheum Dis. 2018 Jan;21(1):36–44.

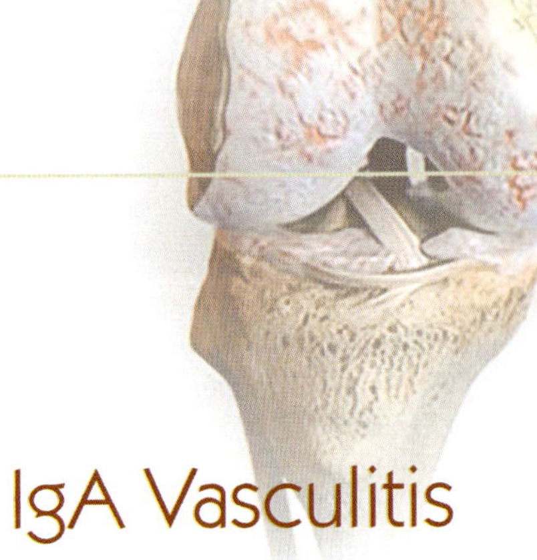

IgA Vasculitis

Col Arun Hegde, Lt col Sankar

INTRODUCTION

Ig A vasculitis also known as HSP (Henoch-Schönlein purpura) earlier, is a small vessel vasculitis characterized by Ig A1 dominant immune deposits in capillaries, venules or arterioles. It predominantly affects children with 90% cases occurring under 10 years of age. It can also be seen in adults with peak incidence in 5th–6th decade. Male to female ratio is 1.5:1. In children, this condition is often preceded by an infection or the use of medications, while in adults, it is typically idiopathic. Clinical features can be diverse ranging from only cutaneous features to systemic involvement with joint symptoms, gastrointestinal and renal involvement. It is generally self-limiting in children but may recur in one-third of patients. Prognosis may be poor in adults, with systemic involvement in up to 75% of the patients.

Clinical Features

i. **Cutaneous:** Rash being the common presenting symptom, seen in almost all patients. It is erythematous petechial or purpuric with subcutaneous edema which is usually symmetrical and appears in crops mostly involving the lower limbs and buttocks. As compared to children, bullae, pustules, necrotic or hemorrhagic purpura can be seen in adults. It is often self-limited.

ii. **Musculoskeletal:** Up to 90% of the patients have musculoskeletal involvement in the form of arthralgia or arthritis. It is usually transient, commonly affecting large joints of lower limb and rarely deformities or erosions are seen.

iii. **Gastrointestinal system:** It is seen in 50–75% of the patients. It may precede or occur after occurrence of rash and symptoms can range from nausea, vomiting, colicky abdominal pain worsening after meals to life threatening complications like GI hemorrhage, bowel angina, perforation and intussusception.

iv. **Renal:** Renal involvement is seen in up to 60% of pediatric population and 85% in adults. It can be asymptomatic, or present with microscopic hematuria (most common), macroscopic hematuria, nephrotic range proteinuria or elevated creatinine in a few patients. Renal involvement predicts the long-term prognosis of the disease. Renal biopsy is indicated in case of persistent hematuria, proteinuria, or azotemia. Regular follow up to 6 months is warranted for patients with renal involvement.

iv. **Other organ systems:** Testicular involvement in form of testicular torsion, central nervous system and peripheral nervous system involvement, lung involvement (diffuse alveolar hemorrhage) and eye involvement have been reported, however these are rare. Ig A vasculitis in adults may be associated with malignancies.

Diagnosis

Ig A vasculitis is primarily a clinical diagnosis. Lab studies may show mild leukocytosis with normal platelet counts. Serum complements are normal, while serum Ig A levels are raised in 50% of the patients. EULAR /Pres/PRINTO criteria are used as a classification criteria used for Ig A vasculitis based on the rash and one out of four of other symptoms (Table 48.1). In challenging or atypical cases, a biopsy of the skin or kidney is recommended, revealing leukocytoclastic vasculitis with predominant IgA deposition on immunofluorescence.

Treatment

Supportive care: Adequate rest, hydration, symptomatic pain relief.

Symptomatic treatment: NSAID is contraindicated in active gastrointestinal bleeding. Mild disease usually resolves with supportive and symptomatic management. Treatment for systemic disease is depicted in Table 48.2.

Severe, Recurrent, or Persistent Disease

In case of severe disease like renal biopsy showing more than 50% crescents, steroid sparing agents like cyclophosphamide, mycophenolate mofetil, cyclosporine or azathioprine to be started along with high dose steroids with tapering. ACE inhibitors or ARBs should be given to all patients with proteinuria.

Table 48.1: EULAR/Pres/PRINTO classification criteria for childhood vasculitis

Criteria	Description
Mandatory	Purpura or petechiae with lower limb predominance
At least one out of four	1. Acute onset diffuse abdominal colicky pain (may include intussusception or GI bleeding) 2. Histology showing leukocytoclastic vasculitis or proliferative glomerulonephritis with predominant IgA deposition. 3. Acute onset arthralgia or arthritis 4. Either proteinuria or hematuria

Table 48.2: Treatment of severe systemic disease

Drug	Dose	Toxicity/ contraindication	Special note
Prednisolone	1–2 mg/kg (max 60–80 g/day)	Hypertension, hyperglycemia	Tapering of steroids over 2 weeks
High dose Intravenous Methylprednisolone	250 mg–1 gm for 3 days	Hypertension, hyperglycemia	In case of active GI bleed or life-threatening organ manifestations
Naproxen	10–20 mg/kg	Can worsen GI bleed or renal function	Contraindicated in active GI bleed or renal dysfunction

B cell depleting agent rituximab and plasma exchange are tried in severe refractory cases without much evidence. Dapsone has been used for severe skin involvement. Renal transplantation is indicated in patients with ESRD.

Prognosis

Majority of the children will have excellent prognosis with more than 90% making complete recovery by 2 years. Up to 2% of the cases can progress to end stage renal disease in children while in adults, it goes up to 13%. Adult patients may have a complicated course. Prognosis in the acute phase is determined by the gastrointestinal complications, while long-term prognosis is determined by severity of renal involvement.

Clinical Snippet

A 19-year-old female presented with multiple purpuric lesions over bilateral lower limbs for 5 days duration. One day after onset of rash, she had colicky pain associated with hematochezia. On examination, there was diffuse tenderness over the abdomen. Investigations revealed mild anemia and leukocytosis with raised acute phase reactants. Her urine microscopic examination showed numerous RBC and 24 hr urinary protein was 600 mg. CECT showed segmental thickening of jejunum and ileum with bowel wall edema and engorgement of the mesenteric vessels. Skin biopsy revealed leukocytoclastic vasculitis with IgA deposits on direct immunofluorescence. She was managed with 1 mg/kg steroids, hydration and analgesics. She showed marked symptomatic improvement over 1 week. Steroids were tapered over 2 weeks and stopped. On follow up her urine routine examination was normal with resolution of proteinuria.

FURTHER READING

1. Xu L, Li Y, Wu X. IgA vasculitis update: Epidemiology, pathogenesis, and biomarkers. Front Immunol. 2022 Oct 3;13:921864. doi: 10.3389/fimmu.2022.921864. PMID: 36263029; PMCID: PMC9574357.
2. Oni L, Sampath S. Childhood IgA Vasculitis (Henoch-Schönlein purpura)—Advances and Knowledge Gaps. Front Pediatr. 2019 Jun 27;7:257.
3. Nidhi Goel, J Sankar, Soham Sen, Manisha Singh, Pradeep Kumar, Sreenivasa S Iyengar, et al. Occlusive retinal vasculitis in IgA vasculitis, *Rheumatology*, 2024; keae337.

Behçet Disease

Sai Sunil B, Sakir Ahmed

INTRODUCTION

Behçet's disease, named after Hulusi Behçet who first described it in 1924, is an inflammatory disorder primarily found along the ancient 'Silk Road', which connects the Mediterranean, Middle East, and Far East. This multisystem disease features a range of symptoms that flare and remit over time. It shares similarities with autoimmune and auto inflammatory disorders.

Pathogenesis

Genetics and epigenetic changes lead to hyperactivity of neutrophils and M1-type differentiation of monocytes/macrophages as well as type 1 helper T cell (Th1) or less prominently Th17 type polarization of adaptive immune response, these inflammatory changes been suggested to play a role in endothelial activation, production of neutrophil extracellular traps (NETs), and thrombotic tendency.

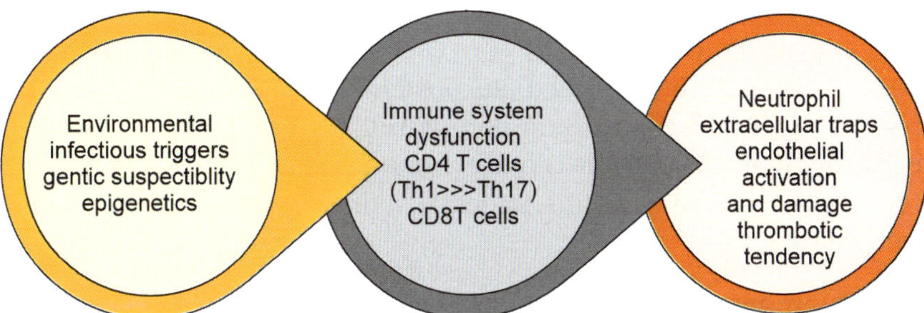

Fig. 49.1: Pathogenesis of Behçet

Putative infectious triggers may be those from *Streptococcus sanguinis, Mycobacterium tuberculosis*, or herpes simplex virus.

Genetic Factorst

HLA genes	Non HLA
HLA-B 51 strong genetic risk factor	STAT4, IL23R–IL12RB2 IL10,22 IL1A, IL1B
MIC-A, HLA-C, 23 HLA-B*27 and HLA-A*26	TNF24, ERAP1, CCR1 and CCR3)

Clinical Features

Oral Ulcers

- Painful round or oval mucosal erosions, on the lips, gingiva, cheeks, and tongue, with a necrotic base surrounded by erythema, heal without scarring, occur early in disease course.

Genital Ulcers

- Occur in 65–75% of patients mostly of the scrotum or labia, are similar to oral ulcers, but larger and deeper which heals slowly, often scars.
- Rarely seen on the shaft of penis, cervix, or vagina.

Cutaneous Lesions

- Acne like lesions, papulopustular lesions on the face, chest and extremities
- Erythema nodosum, pseudofolliculitis-like lesions on the lower limbs (common in women)

Pathergy Test

- Assessing skin hyper-reactivity, can aid in the diagnosis, intradermal skin prick test, some concern that a blunt needle increases the frequency of a positive test and corticosteroids may cause false negative results.

Articular Involvement

- Recurrent asymmetric mono-/oligo-arthritis, or arthralgia, usually at the lower extremities, non-deforming arthritis,
- Around 10% of patients may also manifest with inflammatory back pain, enteropathy and, less frequently, sacroiliitis.

Ocular Involvement

- Common in male often with in first 2–3 years after diagnosis
- Includes uveitis (anterior, intermediate, posterior, or pan uveitis).
- The most common lesions-bilateral non-granulomatous posterior lesions and pan uveitis. Isolated anterior uveitis is less common.
- Other eye issues—retinal vasculitis, ischemia, retinal or vitreous hemorrhage, retinitis, macular edema.

Vascular Involvement

- Common in males, usually in the early disease course.
- The most common are superficial and deep vein thrombosis involving the upper or lower limbs, eventually leading to post-thrombotic syndrome.
- Atypical sites—inferior and superior vena cava, the hepatic veins with Budd-Chiari syndrome, the portal vein, the cerebral venous sinuses thrombosis
- Arterial involvements are frequent with aneurysms involving the peripheral, visceral, and pulmonary arteries.

Hughes-Stovin syndrome: Coexistence of arterial pulmonary aneurysms and venous thrombosis (variant of the vascular Behçet)

Neurological involvement

- Also know as neuro-Behçet's syndrome, typically occurs about 5 years post-diagnosis.
  - Most commonly, the parenchymal region is involved, including the brainstem, telencephalic-diencephalic junction, and basal ganglia, but the spinal cord is less frequently involved. It occurs in two forms—**cute** form-present with fever and high CSF cell count
  - **Chronic** progressive form manifest with ataxia, dementia, sphincter disturbances, and confusion,
- **MRI brain:** Large and extensive lesions and isolated brainstem atrophy

Gastrointestinal

- Symptoms vary from asymptomatic or mild abdominal discomfort to severe pain, with ulcers mainly in the terminal ileocecal region

Complications: Hemorrhage or perforation, can occur in the most severe instances.

Prevalence of Clinical Features

Clinical Feature	Prevalence
Mucocutaneous	95%
Articular involvement,	50–80%
Ocular involvement	50%
Vascular involvement	40%
Neurological involvement	5%
Gastrointestinal	40–60% in Japan, UK

Diagnosis

International Criteria for Behçet Disease

Point score system: Scoring 4 indicates diagnosis of Behçet disease

Sign or Symptom	Points
Ocular lesion	2
Genital aphthosis	2
Oral aphthosis	2
Skin lesions	1
Neurologic manifestations	1
Vascular manifestations	1
Positive pathergy test	1

- Sensitivity 97 6% (95% credible interval 96·9–98·2), specificity 90·8% (89·4–92·1)

Japanese Criteria

Major Symptoms	Minor Symptoms
Recurrent aphthous oral ulcers	Arthritis
Skin lesions	Intestinal ulcers

(Contd.)

(Contd.)

Major Symptoms	Minor Symptoms
Ocular inflammation	Epididymitis
Genital ulcers	Vascular lesions Neuropsychiatric disease
Fulfils criteria:	Patients with all four major symptoms during the clinical course
"Incomplete Behcet"	Three major symptoms Two major and two minor symptoms Typical recurrent ocular inflammation and one or more major symptoms Typical recurrent ocular inflammation and two minor symptoms

International Study Group Criteria

Recurrent major, minor aphthous, or herpetiform oral ulceration, which recurred at least three times over a 12-month period + two manifestations among recurrent genital, ocular, or skin lesions, or positive pathergy test.

Treatment

Manifestation	Recommended treatment	Recommended treatment	Refractory cases
Mucocutaneous	Topical/low dose corticosteroids +/– colchicine →	• Colchicine • Apremilast • azathioprine • Anti-TNF-α	• Thalidomide • IL-1 inhibitors • Secukinumab
Articular	Intra-articular/low dose corticosteroids →	• Azathioprine • Anti TNF-α • Apremilast	• Apremilast • Anakinra • Tofacitinib • Secukinumab
Ocular	Systemic high-dose corticosteroids or topical or intraocular corticosteroids →	• Azathioprine • Cyclosporine • Anti-TNF-α	• Tocilizumab • IL-1 inhibitor
Venous involvement	Corticosteroids Anticoagulants* →	• Azathioprine • Cyclophosphamide • Anti-TNF-α	• Interferon alfa • Cyclosporine
Arterial involvement	Systemic high-dose corticosteroids →	• Cyclophosphamide • Anti-TNF-α • Azathioprine	• Tocilizumab
Neurological	Systemic high-dose corticosteroids →	• Azathioprine • Anti-TNF-α • Cyclophosphamide	• Mycophenolate mofetil • Tocilizumab
Gastrointestinal	Mesalazine Azathioprine →	• ± Corticosteroids • Anti-TNF-α • Thalidomide	• Methotrexate • Ustekinumab

Treatment: Recommended drugs and side effects outlined in the table

Refractory disease: TNF alpha inhibitors, interferon alpha, IL-1 inhibitors, tocilizumab, tofacitinib and secukinumab, thalidomide are used

Drug	Dose	Side effect or contraindication
Colchicine	1–2 mg /day	Diarrhoea, neuromyotoxicity Levels are affected by drug interaction with cytochrome P45
Apremilast	30 mg BD	Diarrhoea, nausea, headache
Azathioprine	2.5 mg/kg/day	Cytopenias
Mycophenolate mofetil	2–3 g/day	Cytopenias
Cyclosporine	3–5 mg/kg/day	Avoid in neuro-Behçet's
Tofacitinib	5 mg BD/11mg OD	Herpes zoster, transaminitis, to be cautious in patient with CV risk factors
Methotrexate	15–25 mg/week	Mucositis/cytopenia/deranged LFT
Thalidomide	50–100 mg/day	Teratogenicity, peripheral neuropathy

Prognosis

- Male sex and early onset are associated with worse disease outcomes.
- The prognosis varies according to ethnicity and the type of disease involvement.
- Mucocutaneous lesions are of minor clinical severity but have a major impact on quality of life.
- Ocular, neurological, and vascular manifestations are the major causes of morbidity.
- Ocular lesions, can lead to visual impairment or loss in 10–20% of patients.
- Vascular Behçet and neuro-Behçet are the leading causes of disability and mortality.

FURTHER READING

1. Lavalle S, Caruso S, Rorti R, Gagliano C, Cocuzza S, Lavia, et al. Behçet Disease, Pathogenesis, Clinical features and Treatment Approaches: A comprehensive Review, Medicine (Kaunas), 2024 Mar 29;60(4):562.

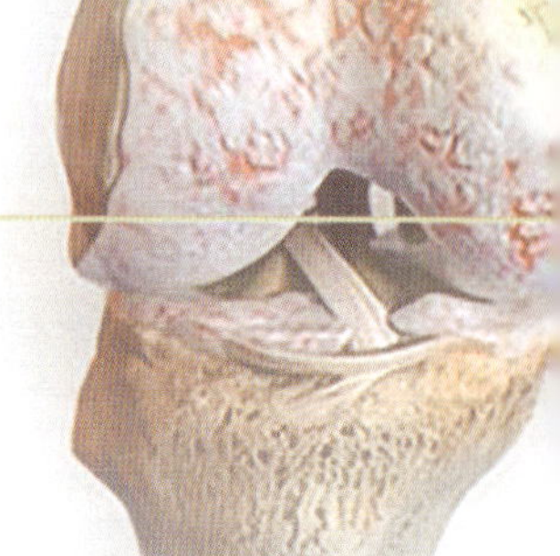

Hypersensitivity Vasculitis

Tejaswee, PD Rath

INTRODUCTION

"Hypersensitivity vasculitis" has been used to refer to a vasculitis of small blood vessels of the skin that is secondary to an immune response or hypersensitivity reaction to an often-unidentifiable exogenous substance.

Also named under two categories in Chapel Hill consensus:

- **Cutaneous leukocytoclastic angiitis** under a newly created category of *Single-organ vasculitis*, consistent with the idea that hypersensitivity has a predilection for the skin.
- **Drug induced immune complex vasculitis**—under a new category of *vasculitis associated with probable etiology*.

   Pathologically characterised by IC deposition in capillaries, postcapillary venules, and arterioles.

   Inciting factor is not detected in around one-third to one-half of patients who are designated as idiopathic CSVV.

Clinical Features

The typical history for a drug-induced hypersensitivity vasculitis is the occurrence of clinical symptoms approximately 7 to 14 days after starting a new medication. Major clinical findings include *palpable purpura* (0.3 to 1 cm diameter) and/or *petechiae* (purpuric lesions less than 3 mm in diameter) that are nonblanching. Sometimes these lesions coalesce, ulcerate, or are surrounded by hemorrhagic bullae. Urticarial lesions can also be observed. Skin lesions are often most prevalent on the lower legs and other dependent areas.

Additional findings:

- Fever
- Malaise
- Myalgias/arthralgias
- Arthritis
- Abdominal pain
- Lymphadenopathy

Drug-induced hypersensitivity vasculitis begin to resolve within days of removal of the offending agent.

Rarely, glomerulonephritis, interstitial nephritis, kidney impairment and varying degrees of hepatocellular injury have all been described. Lung, heart, and central nervous system involvement are less commonly reported.

In cases of immune complex-mediated vasculitis when the inciting agent persists, such as in hepatitis C-related cryoglobulinemic vasculitis, lupus erythematosus, or rheumatoid arthritis, chronic vasculitis can be observed, with waxing and waning lesions or persistent lesions of different ages.

Diagnosis

Clinical findings and by the history of an offending drug or infection (Box 50.1).

Exclude disease in organs other than the skin, the identification of which would implicate another form of vasculitis. Drugs may act as haptens to stimulate an immune response. Drugs like penicillin's, cephalosporins, sulphonamides, loop and thiazide type diuretics, phenytoin, and allopurinol have been most often implicated. Infections such as hepatitis B or C virus, chronic bacteraemias (e.g, infective endocarditis, infected shunts), HIV and severe acute respiratory syndrome Coronavirus 2 (SARS-CoV-2) infections and vaccinations may also be associated with CSVV.

Laboratory Findings

- Mild leucocytosis
- Low serum complement levels, particularly C3 and C4
- Elevated inflammatory markers, such as ESR and CRP.
- Positive culture or serology (e.g, hepatitis C virus) of an infectious agent associated with hypersensitivity vasculitis
- Hematuria, proteinuria, and cellular casts in patients with kidney involvement

Biopsy

Pattern of cutaneous pathology and immunology is highly sensitive to the timing of the biopsy and the age of the lesion, with the lesions between 24 to 48 hours old preferred for biopsy.

Core histological features on biopsy are **infiltration with polymorphonuclear neutrophils in and around the vessel walls,** with signs of activation, degranulation, and death of neutrophils illustrated by **leukocytoclasia (nuclear dust);** evidence of tissue damage (extravasated red blood cells, damaged endothelial cells, and occasionally

---

Box 50.1: American College of Rheumatology 1990 Criteria for the Classification of Hypersensitivity Vasculitis

- Age >16 years
- Use of a possible offending medication in temporal relation to symptoms
- Palpable purpura
- Maculopapular rash
- Biopsy of a skin lesion showing neutrophils around an arteriole or venule

*The presence of **three or more criteria** has a sensitivity of 71% and specificity of 84% for the diagnosis of hypersensitivity vasculitis*

necrosis of skin appendages); and **fibrinoid necrosis**. DIF may show C3, IgM, IgG, IgA deposition.

Treatment

Removal of the inciting agent is the most critical therapy for hypersensitivity vasculitis when the likely agent can be identified. Infection-associated hypersensitivity vasculitis, treatment should be aimed at the underlying infection.

Rest, leg elevation, compression stockings, simple analgesics and oral antihistamines are enough. Severe or persistent cutaneous disease, drugs such as colchicine, antihistamines, NSAIDs, and/or dapsone may be helpful. Immunosuppressive therapy with glucocorticoids or cytotoxic agents should be reserved for the infrequent patient with fulminant or progressive disease or with serious end-organ involvement.

Drug Name	Dose	Toxicity/Contraindications	Special Notes
Prednisolone	0.5 mg/kg/day (20–40 mg)	Caution in uncontrolled DM, HTN	Taper over 3–6 weeks
Colchicine	0.6 mg twice daily	Caution with renal or hepatic impairment or who are taking a P-glycoprotein (P-gp) inhibitor or cytochrome P450 3A4 (CYP3A4) inhibitor Gastrointestinal adverse effects, such as diarrhea, nausea, vomiting, and abdominal pain	No response is noted after one week, increasing the dose to 0.6 mg three times per day may be attempted
Dapsone	100 mg once daily	Idiosyncratic agranulocytosis Hypersensitivity syndrome Hepatitis Peripheral motor neuropathy	Avoided in G6PD deficiency due to a high risk for severe hemolytic anemia

Prognosis

Good prognosis as disease being self-limited with spontaneous resolution within two to four weeks. In patients with self-limited disease, new lesion formation usually continues to occur during the first one to two weeks of the disease process. Chronic or recurrent disease occurs in approximately 10 percent of patients. Postinflammatory hyperpigmentation commonly remain after an episode of CSVV.

Clinical Snippet

A 45-year-old, male with no significant past medical history was started on a sulphonamide antibiotic for urinary tract infection.

5 days after starting the antibiotic, the patient notices:
- Fever
- Painful, erythematous rash on the arms and legs
- Joint pain
- Mild abdominal discomfort

O/E: Rash consists of palpable purpura, particularly on dependent areas (legs and buttocks). Mild arthralgia is noted in the wrists and knees. No signs of systemic infection.

Diagnostic workup: Elevated inflammatory markers (CRP, ESR). Skin biopsy shows leukocytoclastic vasculitis (Fig. 50.1A and B), confirming the diagnosis.

Management: The sulphonamide is discontinued immediately. He was started on corticosteroids to reduce inflammation. Follow-up shows improvement of symptoms and rash resolution over the next few weeks.

This case highlights how a drug reaction can lead to hypersensitivity vasculitis, with characteristic skin findings and systemic symptoms.

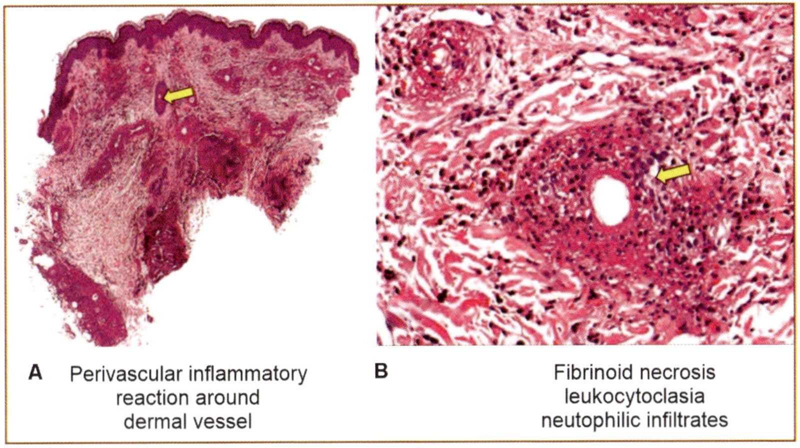

Fig. 50.1A and B: Leukocytoclastic vasculitis

FURTHER READING

1. Hochberg MC, editor. Rheumatology. 8th ed. Philadelphia: Elsevier; 2023.
2. Cabral D, Morishita K. Hypersensitivity vasculitis in children. In: UpToDate [Internet]. Waltham (MA): UpToDate; 2023.

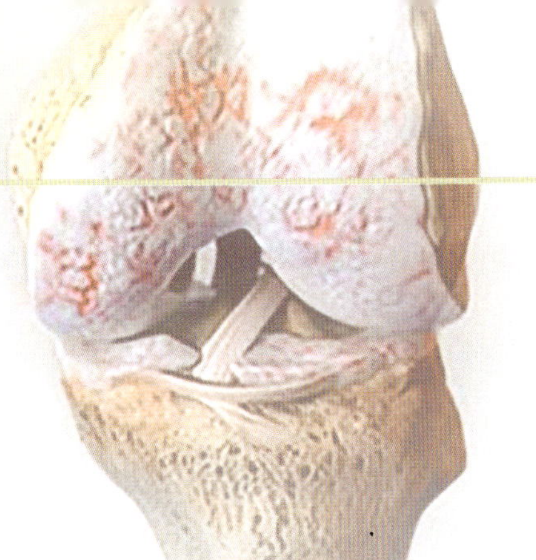

Rheumatology in Special Conditions

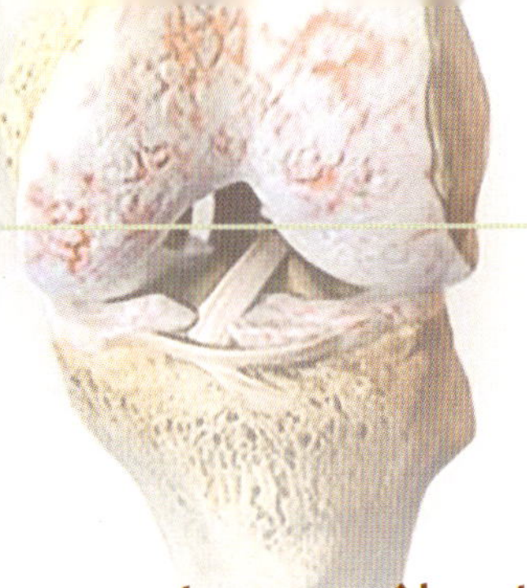

Juvenile Idiopathic Arthritis

Gummadi Anjani

INTRODUCTION

Juvenile idiopathic arthritis (JIA) is the most common rheumatic disease in children. It is a heterogenous group of disorders comprising of varied types of arthritis. The exact cause of JIA is not known, but it involves a combination of genetic, environmental, and immunological factors.

Definition

Arthritis of unknown etiology affecting children younger than 16 years and persisting for 6 weeks or longer with exclusion of other causes of joint inflammation.

Clinical Features

Children with arthritis can have subtle symptoms at onset like stiffness of joints with a limp in early morning or after prolonged rest. Involved joints are often swollen, warm to touch, painful on movement and can have limited range of movements. Infants and toddlers may not be able to express pain and may manifest as irritability in morning, or avoid activities and have regression of achieved milestones. Any number of joints can be involved in JIA. Axial involvement usually sets in later. The number and pattern of joint involvement points to certain diagnosis. If unrecognised, chronic joint damage leads to deformities and limb length discrepancies.

Extra-articular Manifestations

JIA can affect various organs and tissues beyond the joints:
- Fever: Systemic JIA, macrophage activation syndrome
- Skin: Evanescent salmon pink rash in SJIA; psoriasis with nail changes-pitting, onycholysis; rheumatoid nodules
- Ocular involvement: Uveitis of pain and redness of eye
- Hepatosplenomegaly, lymphadenopathy
- Serositis: Pericarditis, pleuritis

Classification of JIA

International League of Associations for Rheumatology Classification

International League of Associations for Rheumatology classifies JIA into 7 subtypes with distinct phenotypes, genetic predispositions, pathophysiology, laboratory findings, disease course, and prognosis.

Category	Clinical feature	Characteristic features/ complications
Systemic JIA	Arthritis Extra-articular manifestation: fever, rash, hepatosplenomegaly, lymphadenopathy, serositis (pericarditis, pleuritis)	Fever is often associated with characteristic rash which is evanescent, salmon-coloured; most commonly over the trunk and proximal extremities Macrophage activation syndrome
Oligoarthritis	≤4 joints	ANA positive Young girls Highest risk of asymptomatic anterior uveitis Need screening for uveitis
Polyarthritis (RF–positive)	≥5 joints Symmetric polyarthritis of small and large joints	Similar to adult rheumatoid arthritis Poor prognosis—deformities, cervical spine involvement
Polyarthritis (RF negative)	≥5 joints	Risk of uveitis
Psoriatic arthritis	Arthritis and psoriasis OR Arthritis and at least 2 of the 3: Dactylitis; nail pitting, onycholysis or psoriasis in a 1st-degree relative	Psoriasis might not manifest at the time of onset of arthritis
Enthesitis related arthritis	Asymmetric arthritis, lower extremity arthritis, enthesitis Adolescent boys	HLA B27 positive- acute symptomatic uveitis
Undifferentiated arthritis	Arthritis that fulfills criteria in no category or in ≥2 of the above categories	

Table 51.1: Categories of International League of Associations for Rheumatology

Pediatric Rheumatology International Trials Organization Classification

Though ILAR classification is accepted worldwhile, a new evidence-based classification model is proposed by the Pediatric Rheumatology International Trials Organization to bring homogenous entities together. According to this, JIA comprises a group of inflammatory disorders that begins before the **18th birthday and includes 5 subtypes**

1. Systemic JIA; 2. RF-positive JIA; 3. Enthesitis/spondylitis-related JIA; 4. Early-onset ANA-positive JIA; and 5. Other

It must be noted that classification criteria are not the same as diagnostic criteria. Classification criteria are mainly meant to have a homogenous population for research purposes.

Diagnosis

Diagnosis of JIA essentially remains clinical, and laboratory investigations usually help to assess the severity of disease activity and extent of organ involvement.

- **Acute-phase reactants:** C-reactive protein (CRP) and erythrocyte sedimentation rate (ESR) and are elevated in active disease.
- **Hemogram:** Platelets are elevated in active disease especially, in SJIA. Falling trend of platelets is marker for evolving macrophage activation syndrome (MAS). Differential counts of WBC will give a clue towards alternate diagnosis, exlymphocytosis in leukemia.
- **Biochemical parameters:** High ferritin, hypofibrinogenemia, high triglyceride and elevated transaminases are seen in SJIA with MAS.
- Testing for **antinuclear antibodies (ANA), human leukocyte antigen (HLA)-B27, and rheumatoid factor (RF)** help to categorize or prognosticate a child with JIA.
- **Imaging:**

  Ultrasound and magnetic resonance imaging (MRI): Useful for detecting early joint inflammation, synovial thickening or proliferation, joint effusion and enthesitis.

  X-rays: Changes are undetectable in an early stage of JIA. Joint space narrowing, bone erosion, periarticular osteopenia and joint subluxation or ankyloses are seen in advanced stages.

Treatment

Early aggressive pharmacotherapy is essential to achieve remission in children with JIA. The commonly used drugs are as follows:

Drug Name	Dose	Toxicity/Special Notes
NSAIDs ex Naproxen	10–20 mg /kg/day in 2 divided doses	GI and renal toxicity; pseudoporphyria
Glucocorticoids	Intra-articular, oral or intravenous depending on subtype of JIA	Not mainstay of treatment Used as bridge therapy, treating flares, severe disease Adverse effects—growth suppression, Cushing syndrome, decreased bone density, immunosuppression
Disease-Modifying Antirheumatic Drug (DMARD) Therapy		
Methotrexate	10–15 mg/m^2 weekly subcutaneous	Folic acid supplementation is must
Sulfasalazine	30–50 mg/kg day in two divided doses	GI intolerance, rash, SJS Not be used in patients with known hypersensitivity to sulfa drugs or salicylates
Leflunomide	<20 kg: 10 mg every other day 20–40 kg: 10 mg daily >40 kg: 20 mg daily, oral	Hepatotoxicity, diarrhea Black box warning for hepatotoxicity
Hydroxychloroquine	<5 mg/kg/day	Retinal toxicity Baseline and annual eye screening

(Contd.)

(Contd.)

Drug Name	Dose	Toxicity/Special Notes
Biological drugs		
Adalimumab	10 kg to <15 kg: 10 mg every other week subcutaneously 15 kg to <30 kg: 20 mg every other week subcutaneously ≥30 kg: 40 mg every other week subcutaneously	TNF inhibitor Infection risk
Tocilizumab	Polyarticular JIA Weight <30 kg: 10 mg/kg: >30 kg: 8 mg/kg every 4 weeks Systemic JIA Weight <30 kg: 12 mg/kg: >30 kg: 8 mg/kg every 2 weeks	IL-6 receptor inhibitor Infection risk, transaminitis, neutropenia, lipid abnormalities
Tofacitinib		Janus kinase inhibitor Infection risk, lipid abnormalities
Anakinra	1–2 mg/kg subcutaneously daily (max 100 mg)	IL1 receptor antagonist Injection site reactions

Hold for suspected bacterial infection, varicella, or measles

Document absence of latent or active tuberculosis and hepatitis B before starting and while on treatment with adalimumab

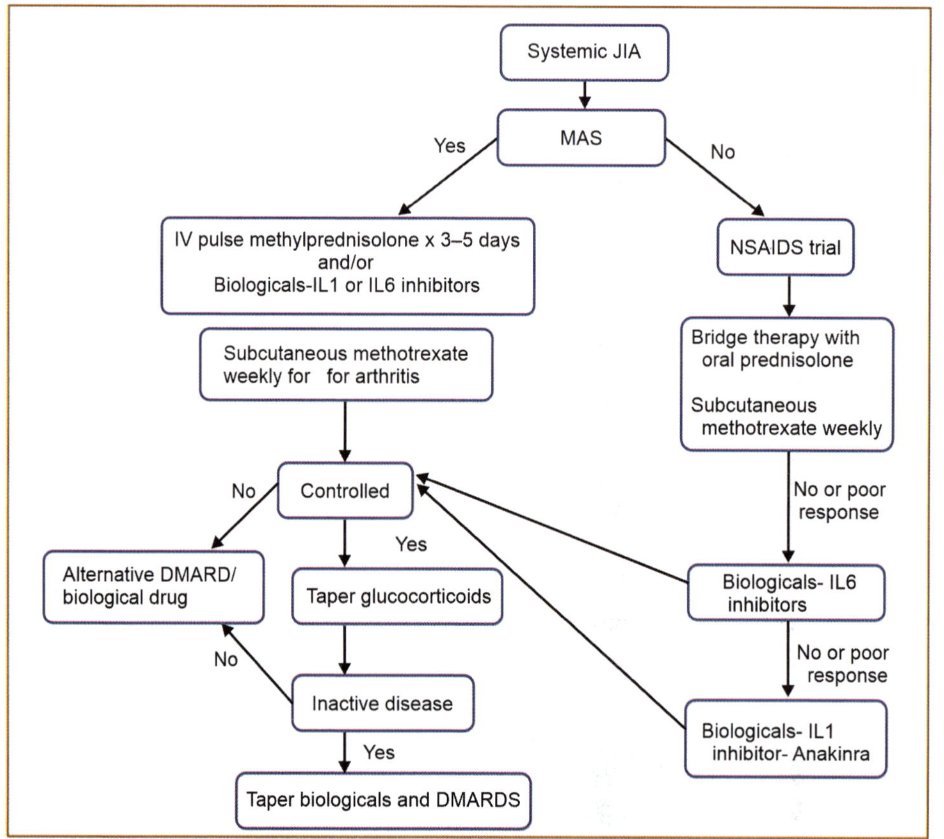

Fig 51.1: Treatment algorithm for systemic JIA

It is advised to use Validated Disease Activity Scores for Assessing Response to Drug

Number and pattern of JIA joints involvement, psoriasis, enthesitis

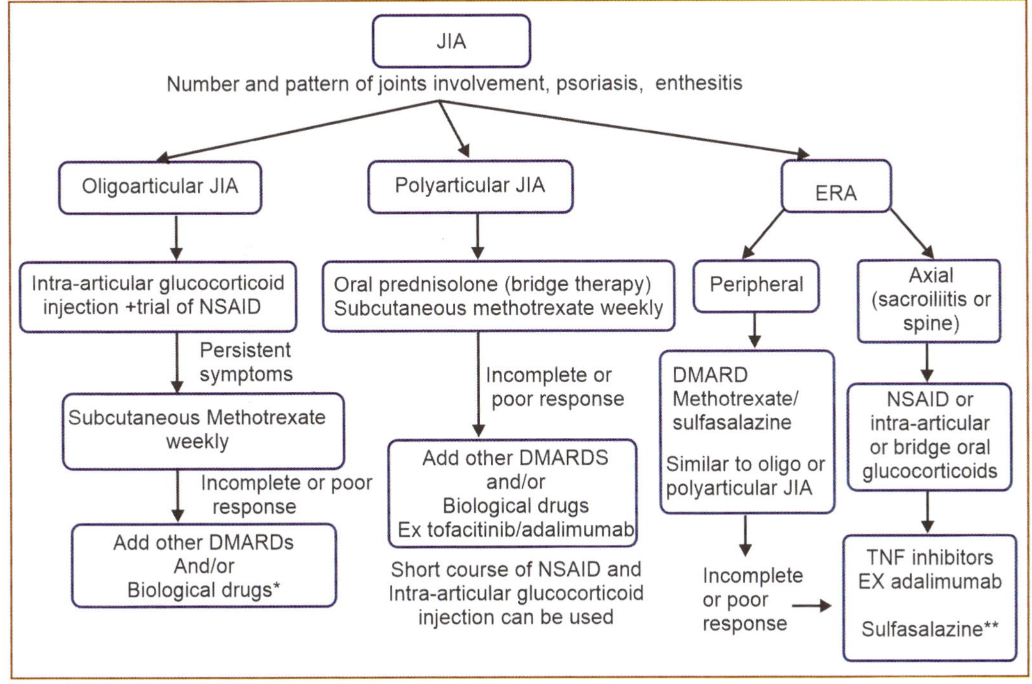

Fig. 51.2: Treatment algorithm for non-systemic JIA.

*presence of poor prognostic factors, high risk joints (ex-cervical spine, hip, wrist) or high disease activity warrant upfront stepping up of therapy or biological drugs
**resource limited settings

Clinical Snippet

Case Presentation

A 4 year-old girl presents with history of right knee pain and swelling × 6 months. She reports morning stiffness lasting more than one hour and parents have noted deformed right knee for last 4 months. There was no history of fever, rash, bone pains, night pains or night awakening. For these symptoms, child was treated elsewhere as septic arthritis and surgery was done. Physical examination reveals a scar on right knee, swelling, tenderness and fixed flexion deformity in the right knee. Also tenderness was noted in the right elbow with deformity.

Investigations

- **ESR:** 50 mm/hr
- **CRP:** 32 mg/L (<1 neg)
- **ANA (Immunoflorescence)** – 2+, speckled pattern

Management Plan

1. Intra-articular triamcinolone injection into right knee.
2. **Initiate methotrexate** at 10–15 mg weekly, subcutaneous with folic acid supplementation.

3. **For faster relief**, can consider low dose glucocorticoids (1–2 mg /kg/day prednisolone equivalent) in tapering doses for 4–6 weeks as a bridge therapy
4. **Eye evaluation for** uveitis every 3–6 months.
5. **Counselling of** parents on the importance of medication adherence and regular monitoring for side effects and disease activity.
6. **Regular follow-up** to adjust therapy based on disease activity and response to treatment.

During follow-up, the primary goals are to taper and eventually discontinue glucocorticoids and to optimize the dose of DMARDs. If a patient does not respond adequately to the current DMARD dose, several strategies can be employed:

1. **Increase the DMARD dose:** Adjusting the dosage to achieve better control of disease activity.
2. **Add another DMARD:** This could include combining DMARDs targeted or biologic DMARDs (for example, Adalimumab) to enhance treatment efficacy.

FURTHER READING

1. Rose E, Petty TRS, Manners P, et al. International league of associations for rheumatology classification of juvenile idiopathic arthritis: second revision, Edmonton, 2001. *J Rheumatol.* 2004;2:390–392.
2. Martini A, Ravelli A, Avcin T, et al. Toward new classification criteria for juvenile idiopathic arthritis: first steps, pediatric rheumatology international trials organization international consensus. *J Rheumatol.* 2019; 46(2):190–97.

Pregnancy and Rheumatology

Vijaya Prasanna Parimi

Autoimmune Rheumatic Diseases and Pregnancy

Autoimmune rheumatic diseases (ARDs) are chronic systemic disorders affecting joints, muscles, and connective tissue, more common in women due to hormonal and genetic factors. Common ARDs in women include rheumatoid arthritis (RA), systemic lupus erythematosus (SLE), antiphospholipid syndrome (APS), and Sjögren's syndrome.

During pregnancy, maternal cardiometabolic adaptations can influence ARD activity, leading to flare-ups or quiescent states, often mistaken for physiological changes. ARDs are linked to adverse pregnancy outcomes (APO) but do not impair fertility. APO may unmask undiagnosed ARD, presenting challenges for patients and their care teams. Successful pregnancies require effective planning, disease control pre-conception, and a multidisciplinary approach.

ARD and Pregnancy: Relationship

ARD can impact pregnancy and pregnancy can affect ARD. Factors such as type of ARD, its activity, medications, and autoantibodies are associated with APO like recurrent pregnancy losses, eclampsia, pre-eclampsia, intrauterine growth restriction (IUGR), premature delivery, intrauterine death (IUD), and stillbirth (Fig 52.1).

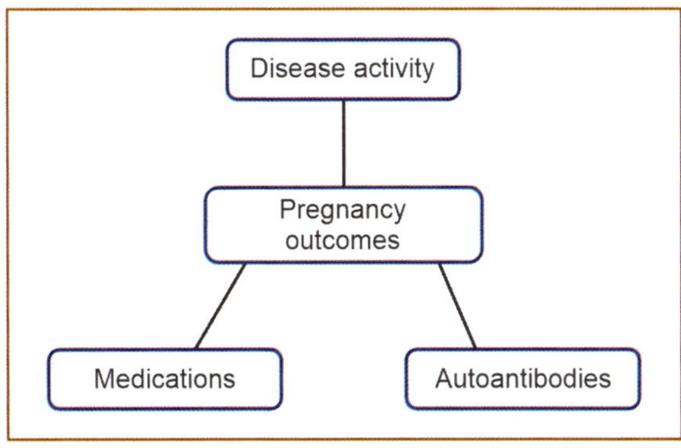

Fig. 52.1: Pregnancy outcomes and risk stratification

Unplanned pregnancies are linked to APO, making it crucial to plan and understand the impact of these disorders. Coordinated medical-obstetrical care, a well-defined management protocol, and a structured neonatal unit are essential to help minimize APO.

Care during the Pre-conceptional Period

Pre-pregnancy counseling is essential for addressing challenges for both mother and fetus. It emphasizes pregnancy planning, disease activity control, safe medications, contraception, antenatal care, lactation, and maternal and neonatal health. Pregnancy timing is critical, with conception recommended during disease remission for 6 to 12 months to reduce adverse outcomes. Women with active lupus nephritis, recent strokes, or severe organ involvement, such as pulmonary hypertension or interstitial lung disease (ILD), should delay or avoid pregnancy due to high risks.

Contraceptive options should align with underlying conditions; progesterone-only methods and intrauterine devices are effective in active lupus. Assisted reproductive techniques and fertility preservation may also be considered. Key antibodies like anti-Ro/SSA and anti-La/SSB require monitoring due to risks of fetal heart block and neonatal lupus. Antiphospholipid antibodies necessitate anticoagulation during pregnancy and postpartum.

Teratogenic drugs, including methotrexate and mycophenolate, must be discontinued and replaced with safer alternatives like hydroxychloroquine, sulfasalazine, and low-dose steroids. Contraception is critical for women on teratogenic medications, while corticosteroids like prednisone are generally safe at doses below 20 mg/day. Male fertility and teratogenicity also warrant attention during pre-conception planning.

Antenatal Care

Pregnancy confirmation necessitates antibody testing, disease assessment, differentiation of physiological pregnancy manifestations from underlying ARD, medication use, fetal heart monitoring, fetal growth assessment, maternal blood pressure monitoring, and regular rheumatologist consultation (Fig. 52.2).

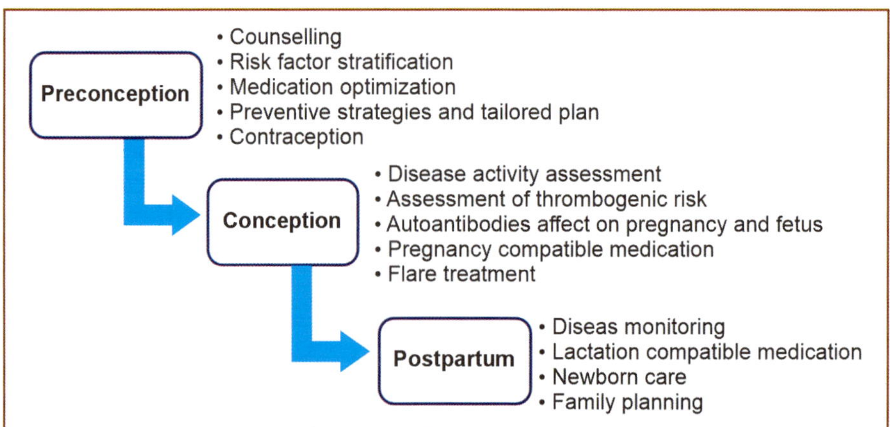

Fig. 52.2: Prenatal, antepartum, and postpartum care in women with autoimmune rheumatological musculoskeletal diseases

Postpartum Care

Pregnant women with ARD face a high risk of postpartum flares. Infants born to women with anti-Ro/SSA and/or anti-La/SSB antibodies may develop neonatal lupus, manifesting as rash, transient cytopenias, and transaminitis. Complete heart block occurs in a small percentage of pregnancies, and anticoagulation must be continued for six weeks postpartum to mitigate the risk of thrombosis, including cerebral venous sinus thrombosis (CVST) and deep vein thrombosis (DVT).

Effect of Pregnancies on Rheumatic Diseases

Pregnancy in lupus and APS is challenging due to high rates of flare-ups and pregnancy loss. Effective treatment reduces the chance of loss, while quiescent SLE patients have fewer flares. Lupus increases thrombosis risk during pregnancy and postpartum. Pre-eclampsia is common, especially in women with hypertension or a history of lupus nephritis, and low-dose aspirin can reduce this risk.

Pregnancy outcomes for women with RA are generally favorable, but disease activity may increase. The use of disease-modifying antirheumatic drugs (DMARDs) can elevate risks of pre-eclampsia and cesarean-section. Stopping medications or active disease before conception increases flare risks.

Pregnancy often worsens ankylosing spondylitis (AS) symptoms like stiffness, tenderness, and pain, but does not increase miscarriage or delivery complications. Non-steroidal anti-inflammatory drugs are used for flares but should be avoided after 32 weeks due to the risk of premature closure of the ductus arteriosus.

Scleroderma disease activity generally remains stable during pregnancy, although Raynaud's phenomenon may improve and gastroesophageal reflux may worsen. Close monitoring is essential, as scleroderma renal crisis is a serious complication. Premature births and fetal death can occur in small vessel vasculitis, Takayasu arteritis, and Behcet's disease.

Long-Term Health Implications of Adverse Pregnancy Outcomes

Pregnancy can significantly affect the long-term health of women with ARD, with some experiencing remission during pregnancy and others having flare-ups postpartum. Management strategies may include medication adjustments, monitoring disease activity, and supporting the mother's physical and emotional well-being. APOs can increase the future risk of cardiovascular diseases in these women.

Management of Pregnancy in ARD

Managing pregnancy in women with ARD requires a multidisciplinary team involving rheumatologists, obstetricians, and neonatologists. Risk stratification should consider the extent of maternal disease, previous APO, and antibody status. Medication management is critical, balancing disease control with fetal safety. A personalized treat-to-target approach is essential for suppressing disease activity and achieving optimal outcomes.

Conclusion

Pregnancy in women with autoimmune rheumatic diseases presents unique challenges. From pre-conception to postpartum, a multidisciplinary approach is crucial to ensure the best outcomes. Achieving disease quiescence before conception and using pregnancy-compatible medications are essential for successful pregnancies.

Table 52.1: Drug safety during pregnancy and lactation

Drug	Preconception	Antenatal	lactation
Prednisolone	Yes	Yes	Yes
Hydroxychloroquine	Yes	Yes	Yes
Methotrexate	No Stop 1–3 months before conception	No	No
Sulphasalazine	Yes	Yes	Yes
Leflunomide	No Cholestyramine wash out required	No	No
Azathioprine	Yes	Yes	Yes
Mycophenolate	No Stop 6 weeks of preconception	No	No
Calcineurin inhibitors (cyclosporine, tacrolimus)	Yes	Yes	Yes
Intravenous immunoglobulin	Yes	Yes	Yes
Biologics	Each medication should be considered separately when making decisions about continuing biologic treatement during pregnancy.		

FURTHER READING

1. Andreoli L, Bertsias GK, Agmon-Levin N, et al. EULAR recommendations for women's health and the management of family planning, assisted reproduction, pregnancy and menopause in patients with systemic lupus erythematosus and/or antiphospholipid syndrome. *Ann Rheum Dis*. 2017;76(3):476-485. doi: 10.1136/annrheumdis-2016-209770.
2. Sammaritano LR. Contraception and preconception counseling in women with autoimmune disease. *Best Pract Res Clin Obstet Gynaecol*. 2020;64:11-23. doi: 10.1016/j.bpobgyn.2019.09.003.

Drugs in Pregnancy and Lactation

Sunitha kayidhi

INTRODUCTION

The decision to use any drug during pregnancy depends on clinical context, severity of disease, risk associated with particular medication and gestational age.

Recommendations for antirheumatic medication use during pregnancy and breastfeeding have been issued by four distinct bodies, ACR2020 (American College of Rheumatology), BSR 2023 (British Society of Rheumatology, EULAR 2016 (European league against rheumatism) and ACOG 2019 (American College of Obstetricians and Gynecologists).

Tables 53.1 through 3 provide an overview of the comparison of these recommendations.

Table 53.1: Anti-rheumatic drugs compatible with pre-conception and pregnancy					
	ACR 2019	*BSR 2016*	*EULAR 2016*	*ACOG 2019*	*Comments*
Hydroxychloro-quine	++	Yes	Compatible	Low risk	Preferably at doses <400 mg/day
Prednisolone/ methylprednsio-lone	++	Yes	Compatible	Low risk	Should be given at least dose possible Intra-articular, intravenous and intramuscular steroids can be given[3]
NSAIDs (Classical)	+	–	Compatible	–	Use in 1st and 2nd trimesters only discontinue in pre-conception if woman has difficulty conceiving 1
NSAIDs (Coxibs)	Not preferred	–	Not compatible	–	Celecoxib is preferable

(Contd.)

(Contd.)

Drug	ACR 2019	BSR 2016	EULAR 2016	ACOG 2019	Comments
Sulfasalazine	++	Yes	Compatible	Low risk	Use folic acid 5 mg in the preconception period and first trimester[2,4] Dosed up to 2 g/day are advisable[3]
Azathioprine/ 6-Mercaptopurine	++	Yes	Compatible	Low risk	Doses up to 2 mg/kg/day are advisable[3]
Colchicine	++	–	–	–	
Tacrolimus	++	Yes	Compatible	–	Monitor blood pressure[1,2] renal function, blood glucose and drug levels[2]
Cyclosporine	++	Yes	Compatible	Low risk	
TNF inhibitors (TNFi) INF, ADA, ETA and GOL	+Continue in 1st and 2nd trimesters Discontinue in 3rd trimester	Yes	INF &ADA can be given up to 20 weeks, ETA up to 30–32 weeks (or throughout pregnancy if needed) GOL-limited evidence to suggest	Low to moderate risk	live vaccines should be avoided in infants until they are 6 months of age in all the TNFi except CZP Women considered to have low risk of disease flare on withdrawal of TNFi in pregnancy could stop INF at 20 weeks, ADA and GOL at 28 weeks, and ETA at 32 weeks so that a full-term infant can have a normal vaccination schedule, with rotavirus vaccination at 8 weeks[2]
Certolizumab	++	Yes	Compatible		
IV immunoglobulin	–	Yes	Compatible	–	

ACR categorises medication into

++ Strongly recommend
+ Conditionally recommend
× Conditionally recommend against
×× Strongly recommend against

ACOG categorises medication into four categories

1. Low risk in pregnancy which can be continued throughout pregnancy.
2. Low risk emerging therapies with developing for use in pregnancy.
3. Intermediate risk with little or no existing data on use.
4. High risk medication generally contraindicated in pregnancy.

Anti-Rheumatic Drugs Considered High Risk in Pregnancy

Drug	ACR	BSR	EULAR	ACOG	Time (in months) to stop medication before planning conception
NOT RECOMMENDED					
Methotrexate	xx	No	Not compatible	High risk	1 month prior[1] 1–3 months prior[2,3]
Leflunomide	xx	No	Not compatible	High risk	Cholestyramine washout if detectable levels are present.[1,2] Pregnancy should be avoided until serum drug levels drop below 0.02 mg/L on two occasions,[2] weeks apart[4]
Mycophenolate mofetyl	xx	No	Not compatible	High risk	>6 weeks before planning conception[1,2]
Thalidomide	xx		–	–	1–3 months prior[1]
Tofacitinib Baricitinib	Unable to suggest due to low evidence	No	Not compatible	–	2 weeks before conception[2]
Apremilast		–		–	

Not recommended except for life or organ threatening maternal disease, where other compatible drugs cannot be used

Drug	ACR	BSR	EULAR	ACOG	Time (in months) to stop medication before planning conception
Cyclophosphamide	Use In 2nd & 3rd trimesters	Throughout pregnancy	In 2nd & 3rd trimesters	Moderate to high risk in the first trimester—use in 2nd & 3rd trimesters	Stop 3 months prior planning conception[1]
Rituximab	+	Yes	Yes	Not studied	• Stop these drugs at conception[1,2]
Tocilizumab	x	Yes	Cannot suggest due to limited evidence	–	If used in third trimester, live vaccines should be avoided in infants until they are 6 months of age
Anakinra Canakinumab	x	Yes		–	
Abatacept	x	Yes		–	• For rituximab, should be aware of risk of B cell depletion and cytopenias in neonate
Belimumab	x	Yes		Not studied	
Secukinumab	x	Yes		–	
Ustekinumab	x	Yes		–	

INF: Infliximab; ADA: Adalimumab; ETA: Etanercept; GOL: Golimumab

Antirheumatic Drugs in Lactation

	ACR	BSR	EULAR	ACOG
HCQS	++	Yes	Compatible	Compatible
Sulfasalazine	++	Yes, in healthy full-term infant only	Compatible	Compatible
Colchicine	++	–	Compatible	–
Azathioprine/6-Mercaptopurine	+	Yes	Compatible	Compatible
Prednisolone	+	Yes	Compatible	Compatible
	Delay breastfeeding for 4 hours for the doses >20 mg/day			Compatible
NSAIDs (classic)	+ Ibuprofen preferred	–	Compatible Celecoxib only in COX -II inhibitors Group	–
Methotrexate	x	No	Not compatible	Not compatible
Lefluonamide	xx	No	Not compatible	Not studied
Mycophenolate mofetil	xx	No	Not compatible	Not studied
Cyclophosphamide	xx	No	Not compatible	Compatible
Rituximab	++		Not compatible	Not studied
Anakinra, belimumab, abatacept, tocilizumab, secukinumab, Ustekinumab	+ Limited data Possible less transfer due to large molecular weight	Yes	Not compatible	Not studied
Tofactinib Baricitinib	Unable to suggest due to less evidence	No	Not compatible	–
Apremilast	May cross placenta due to their small size	–	–	–
Thalidomide	xx	–	–	–
IVIg	–	Yes	Compatible	–

FURTHER READING

1. Sammaritano LR, Bermas BL, Chakravarty EE, et al. 2020 American College of Rheumatology Guideline for the Management of Reproductive Health in Rheumatic and Musculoskeletal Diseases. Arthritis Care Res (Hoboken). 2020;72(4):461-488. doi:10.1002/acr.24130

2. Russell MD, Dey M, Flint J, et al. British Society for Rheumatology guideline on prescribing drugs in pregnancy and breastfeeding: immunomodulatory anti-rheumatic drugs and corticosteroids [published correction appears in Rheumatology (Oxford). 2023 May 2;62(5):2021.

3. Götestam Skorpen C, Hoeltzenbein M, Tincani A, et al. The EULAR points to consider for use of antirheumatic drugs before pregnancy, and during pregnancy and lactation Annals of the Rheumatic Diseases 2016;75:795–810.

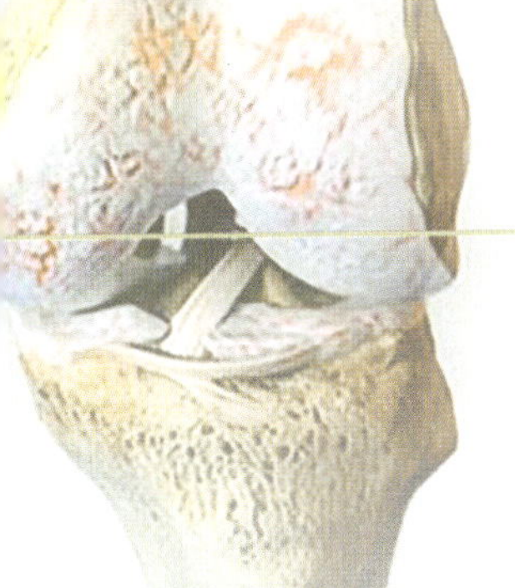

Drugs in Renal Diseases

Jithin Mathew

INTRODUCTION

Renal involvement and renal dysfunction are important manifestations of many systemic autoimmune rheumatic diseases (SARD) like systemic lupus erythematosus ANCA vasculitis, cryoglobulinemic vasculitis, IgA vasculitis, polyarteritis nodosa, secondary renal amyloidosis. The clinical picture may range from nephrotic syndrome to frank nephritic syndrome with reduced glomerular filtration rate. Renal dysfunction may also occur due to co-morbid causes like chronic NSAID abuse, long-standing diabetes or hypertension, renovascular disease, stone disease, etc . The presence of renal dysfunction may necessitate the use or avoidance of certain medicines with careful consideration of dosing schedules to minimize drug-induced adverse effects in patients with underlying rheumatic diseases.

Renal Toxicity due to Drugs used for Managing Rheumatic Conditions

Certain drugs are inherently nephrotoxic by either causing changes in the intra-renal hemodynamics or inducing fibrotic changes in the various renal compartments are given in Table 54.1.

Considerations in Patients with Pre-existing Renal Disease

The renal safety profile of individual classes of drugs and guidance to their use in renal dysfunction are detailed below.

Table 54.1: Nephrotoxic drugs used for managing SARD	
Drug	*Associated Renal Toxicity*
NSAIDs	Chronic use may result in analgesic nephropathy and CKD. Acute use may rarely result in acute interstitial nephritis
Cyclosporine tacrolimus	Calcineurin inhibitors are known to cause both acute and chronic changes in renal function and may rarely even be associated with thrombotic microangiopathy. Acute changes in creatinine are reversal with discontinuation in most cases

a. Conventional DMARDs (Table 54.2).
b. Biological DMARDs (Table 54.3).
c. Small Molecule DMARDs (Table 54.4).
d. Miscellaneous (Table 54.5).

Table 54.2: Use of csDMARDs in patients with SARD and pre-existing renal disease

Drug	Consideration
Methotrexate	Creatinine Clearance (CrCl) <30 ml/min/1.73 m^2-Avoid CrCl-30–60–Use judiciously, reduce dose by 50%, preferable use alternative agents Avoid use in hemodialysis (HD) and peritoneal dialysis (PD) High risk of fatal myelosuppression in patients with reduced GFR as it is excreted primarily through kidneys
Sulfasalazine	Insufficient data to guide use, caution to be exercised if being used, preferable to avoid Low dose <1 gm/day – possibly safe in HD & PD
Leflunomide	Conflicting data, use with caution Mild renal impairment—no dose adjustment needed Moderate-severe renal impairment—contraindicated HD/PD—use with caution
Hydroxychloroquine	Short term treatment—no adjustment needed Long term treatment—dose adjustment required Renal dysfunction may potentiate retino-toxicity and cardiac toxicity
Azathioprine	Crcl >30—no adjustment Crcl 10–30—75–100% of planned dose Crcl <10—50–100% of planned dose
Cyclophosphamide	>30—no adjustment CrCl <30—reduce planned dose by 30% HD—70–75% of planned dose on dialysis days, administer after hemodialysis, allowing at least 12 hours before the next hemodialysis session
Mycophenolate mofetil	No dose adjustment necessary

Table 54.3: Use of csDMARDs in patients with SARD and pre-existing renal disease

Drug	Consideration
Anti-tumor Necrosis factor Alpha agents	Safe and effective in all stages of CKD, no dose adjustment needed. HD/PD—no adjustment needed, non-dialysable Monitor for increased risk of infections on background of CKD
Rituximab	Safe and effective, no dose adjustment needed HD/PD—no adjustment needed, non-dialysable
Tocilizumab	Safe and effective, no dose adjustment needed HD/PD—no adjustment needed, non-dialysable
Anakinra	CrCl 60–<90 ml/min—no dose adjustment needed CrCl 30–<60 ml/min—caution should be exercised CrCl <30 ml/min/dialysis—the administration of recommended therapeutic dose should be considered every other day HD/PD—not dialysable

(Contd.)

(Contd.)

Drug	Consideration
Abatacept	No data available to guide usage
IL 17 inhibitor (Secukinumab/ ixekizumab)	No formal data Use is possibly safe based on isolated case reports with no dosing adjustment needed even on HD/PD
IL- 12/23 inhibitors Ustekinumab	No formal data Use is possibly safe based on isolated case reports with no dosing adjustment needed even on HD/PD

Table 54.4: Targeted Synthetic DMARDs in patients with SARD and pre-existing renal disease

Drug	Consideration
Tofacitinib	CrCl >30—no adjustment needed CrCl <30—reduce dose to 5 mg od HD—on HD days, administer after HD
Baricitinib	CrCl >60—no adjustment needed CrCl 30–60—reduce dose by 50% CrCl <30—avoid HD/PD—avoid
Upadacitinib	CrCl >30—no adjustment CrCl 15–30—caution (15 mg/day) CrCl <15—avoid HD/PD—avoid

Table 54.5: Miscellaneous drugs in pre-existing renal disease

Drug	Consideration
Glucocorticoids	No dose adjustment needed Consider infection risk in patients with CKD
Tramadol	CrCl >30—no adjustment CrCl <30—max 200 mg/day; Increase dosing interval to 12 hours

Conclusion

Using rheumatic drugs in patients with renal disease demands a careful individualized approach to mitigate potential nephrotoxicity and adverse effects. Renal involvement in systemic autoimmune diseases, such as lupus and vasculitides, alongside renal dysfunction from chronic conditions like hypertension or diabetes, requires thoughtful drug selection and dosing adjustments. Conventional DMARDs, such as methotrexate and cyclophosphamide, require dose adjustments based on renal function, while biologic DMARDs generally exhibit a safer renal profile, with most being usable without significant dosing changes even in patients on dialysis. However, newer small-molecule DMARDs such as tofacitinib and baricitinib necessitate careful dosage modulation in cases of reduced creatinine clearance

FURTHER READING

1. Tyczyńska KM, Augustyniak-Bartosik H, Świerkot J. Rheumatoid arthritis - medication dosage in chronic kidney disease. Reumatologia. 2023;61(6):481–491.

2. Schiff MH, Whelton A. Renal toxicity associated with disease-modifying antirheumatic drugs used for the treatment of rheumatoid arthritis. Semin Arthritis Rheum. 2000 Dec;30(3):196-208

3. Yoshimura Y, Yamanouchi M, Mizuno H, et al. Efficacy and safety of first-line biological DMARDs in rheumatoid arthritis patients with chronic kidney disease. *Annals of the Rheumatic Diseases* 2024;83:1278–1287.

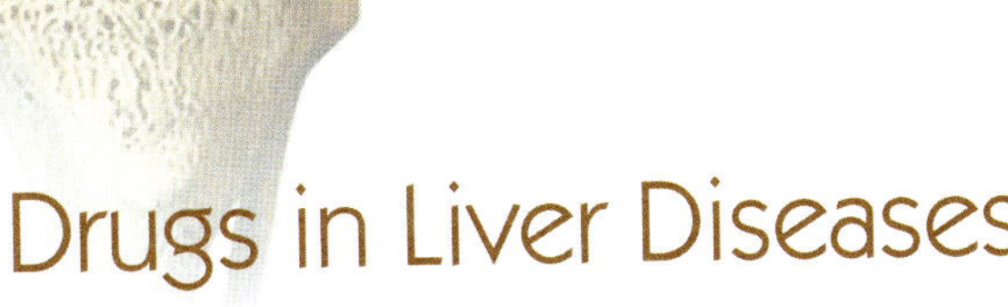

Drugs in Liver Diseases

Shruti Sripathi

INTRODUCTION

Liver involvement and its dysfunction can occur in as much as 43% of patients with rheumatological diseases. Liver involvement in rheumatological disorders may range from asymptomatic elevation of transaminases or cholestatic enzymes to the development of cirrhosis. The commonest etiologies reported to cause liver abnormalities are drug-induced liver injury (DILI), concomitant viral hepatitis, fatty liver disease and autoimmune liver disease.

Drug-induced Liver Injury

Rheumatic diseases are treated using a range of medications, most of which transiently increase liver enzymes. Drug-induced liver damage can sometimes progress to advanced liver diseases, such as fibrosis, cirrhosis, and fulminant liver failure. Some medications directly affect the liver, while some indirectly induce the reactivation of latent infections or autoimmune diseases.

Various drugs in managing CTDs and their respective liver involvement

Drug	Severity
Non-steroidal anti-inflammatory drugs	Liver injury is usually mild and improves with treatment discontinuation
Methotrexate	Causes mild elevation of aminotransferases in up to 13% occasionally leading to cirrhosis. (BMI, alcohol consumption and lack of folic acid supplementation may play a role) If the increase in aminotransferases >3 × upper limit of normal (ULN), MTX should be discontinued. If liver test abnormalities persist, a liver biopsy ought to be performed. In case of normalization of aminotransferases, MTX may be restarted at a lower dose
Leflonamide	Causes asymptomatic aminotransferase elevation in up to 20% of patients. Not recommended for use in patients with pre-existing liver disease or those with baseline ALT >2 times ULN
Tumor necrosis factor-alpha inhibitors	Causes asymptomatic aminotransferase elevation of 2 to 3 times the upper limit of normal in 37–42% of patients. Can trigger autoimmune hepatitis, hepatitis B reactivation.

(Contd.)

(Contd.)

Drug	Severity
Tocilizumab	Causes transient elevation of liver enzymes but it is asymptomatic and short-lived.
Rituximab	Reactivation of hepatitis B in patients who have been tested HBsAg-positive and HBsAg-negative/HBc-positive patients and thus, requires additional antiviral prophylaxis treatment.
Tofacitinib	Hepatitis B reactivation can lead to severe acute liver injury.
Steroids	High-dose steroids can lead to hepatitis B reactivation. HBsAg positive with DNA>2000 IU/ml need antiviral treatment whereas those with DNA<2000 need prophylaxis if using moderate to high dose steroid Antiviral prophylaxis is necessary in patients with HBsAg negative but hepatitis B core and HBV DNA positivity.

Check CBP, creatinine/calculated GFR, ALT and AST every:

- Monthly for three months
- Thereafter monitor at least every 2–3 months.
- More frequent monitoring is appropriate in patients at higher risk of toxicity

Drugs in Special Conditions

Non-alcoholic Fatty Liver Disease (NAFLD)

Methotrexate is recommended over alternative DMARDs for DMARD-naive patients with NAFLD, normal liver enzymes and liver function tests and no evidence of advanced liver fibrosis (stage 3 or 4). Non-invasive testing to diagnose and stage liver fibrosis should be considered in patients before initiating methotrexate. In addition, more frequent monitoring should be performed in this patient population.

Hepatitis B Infection

Risk of HBV reactivation with various drugs

Drug	Chronic HBV infection (HBsAg positive)	Resolved HBV infection (HBsAg negative, anti-HBc positive)
Rituximab	Very High	Moderate
High-dose corticosteroids (over 20 mg prednisolone or equivalent)	High	Low
Anti-TNF	Moderate	Low
IL-6 inhibitors	Moderate	Low
IL-17 inhibitors	Moderate	Low
Abatacept	Moderate	Low
JAK inhibitors	Moderate	Low
Cyclophosphamide	Moderate	Low
Mycophenolate mofetil	Low	Low
Methotrexate	Low	Low
Leflonamide	Low	Low
Sulfasalazine	Low	Low

Although reported cases of HBV reactivation vary, very high risk are considered to be >20%, high is 11–20%, moderate between 1 and 10% and low<1%.

Screening for hepatitis B virus must include HBsAg, anti-HBc IgM and IgG and anti-HBs before starting immunosuppressive medication.

Prophylactic antiviral therapy is strongly recommended over frequent monitoring of viral load and liver enzymes alone for patients initiating rituximab who are hepatitis B core antibody positive (regardless of hepatitis B surface antigen status)

Prophylactic antiviral therapy is strongly recommended over frequent monitoring alone for patients initiating any bDMARD or tsDMARD who are hepatitis B core antibody positive and hepatitis B surface antigen positive.

Frequent monitoring alone of viral load and liver enzymes is recommended over prophylactic antiviral therapy for patients initiating a bDMARD other than rituximab or a tsDMARD who are hepatitis B core antibody positive and hepatitis B surface antigen negative patients.

Hepatitis C Infection

Hepatitis C reactivation following immunosuppressive therapy in contrast to HBV reactivation is rare but when occurs the mortality and morbidity are the same.

Before initiating immunosuppressive drugs, patients should be screened for chronic HCV and closely monitored for liver enzymes as well as HCV viral load. In patients with chronic HCV, ACR recommends that etanercept may be administered in patients with acute or chronic HCV with severe liver damage (Child-Pugh classification B or C), biological agents should be avoided.

Chronic Liver Disease

Chronic liver disease	<ul><li>MTX is contraindicated</li><li>Leflonamide and sulfasalazine are contraindicated in child C status</li><li>Preferable to avoid leflunomide in mild and moderate impairment (Child A and B)</li><li>Biologics contraindicated in child B and C.</li><li>Half dosing of tofacitinib can be used with caution in child B status.</li><li>NSAIDs like diclofenac can precipitate hepatorenal syndrome.</li></ul>	<ul><li>HCQ is safe</li><li>SSZ safe in child A status</li><li>Cyclosporin A can be given</li></ul>

Conclusion

Abnormalities in liver function tests are common in patients with rheumatic diseases. Careful monitoring of liver enzymes is crucial to detect liver diseases and prevent their evolution to chronic liver disease and cirrhosis. Screening for viral hepatitis B and C is necessary to avoid an aggravation of chronic infection and re-activation of latent infection.

FURTHER READING

1. Fraenkel L, Bathon JM, England BR, et al. 2021 American College of Rheumatology Guideline for the Treatment of Rheumatoid Arthritis. *Arthritis Rheumatol.* 2021;73(7):1108–23.
2. Loomba R, Liang TJ. Hepatitis B reactivation associated with immune suppressive and biological modifier therapies: current concepts, management strategies, and future directions. Gastroenterology 2017; 152:1297–1309.

Surgical Interventions in Rheumatology

Sreejitha KS

The treatment of rheumatologic illnesses has seen massive advances in the preceding decades resulting in early pharmacological and biologic therapies targeting the molecular pathogenesis of disease. This reduces joint damage and deformities pushing surgical treatment to the backseat. This chapter discusses the relevance of surgery in the current era, along with the perioperative treatment modifications in a patient with rheumatological disease.

1. **Rheumatoid arthritis:** The main goals of surgery are pain relief, correction of instability, reconstruction of damaged structures and cosmetic correction. These come into play in case of failed pharmacological management, long-standing disease or non-compliance with treatment.

   The commonly used procedures are:

   i. **Synovectomy:** Removal of inflamed synovium from joints (arthrosynovectomy) or tendons (tenosynovectomy).

   ii. **Arthrodesis:** Articular cartilage is removed and joint surfaces fixed in chronic painful, unstable joints where mobility cannot be salvaged, resulting in a painless fixed joint.

   iii. **Arthroplasty:** Reconstruction of joints with prosthetic or endogenous materials.

   iv. Repair of damaged tendons, correction of soft tissue malpositions, etc.

   The various procedures in different joints are compiled in Table 56.1.

Table 56.1: Various procedures in different joints			
Joint	*Indications for surgery*	*Procedures*	*Outcomes*
Cervical spine Thoracolumbar spine	Atlantoaxial dislocation with impending spinal cord injury Intractable pain Vertebral collapse	Arthrodesis- fusion of base of skull to C1/atlantoaxial fusion +/- decompression C1 laminectomy Vertebroplasty/kyphoplasty	Pain relief up to 80% Pain relief, improved function

(Contd.)

(Contd.)

Joint	Indications for surgery	Procedures	Outcomes
Shoulder	Intractable pain Severe limitation of movement Rotator cuff tear	Synovectomy (less damaged joints) Prosthetic joint arthroplasty total arthroplasty or hemiprosthesis-in damaged joints Rotator cuff repair	Pain relief Additional benefit to neck and elbow
Elbow	Unresponsive pain Limitation of movement Instability	Synovectomy with radial head removal Total elbow replacement	Pain relief (60%) Pain relief (90%), improved flexion
Wrist	Pain (impending) tendon rupture Malalignment		
Elbow	Unresponsive pain Limitation of movement Instability	Synovectomy with radial head removal Total elbow replacement	Pain relief (60%) Pain relief (90%), improved flexion
Wrist	Pain (impending) tendon rupture Malalignment	Synovectomy Rebalancing of extensors Arthrodesis Prosthetic joint (Radiocarpal) reconstruction	Pain relief
Hand	Tendon rupture Loss of function from deformities	Tenosynovectomy Arthrodesis Tendon repair/ transfer/ graft Prosthetic reconstruction	Improved hand function Pain relief and stability
Hip	Pain and limitation of movement, limb shortening	Arthroplasty	Pain relief and improved mobility
Knee	Pain Reduced mobility	Synovectomy Arthroplasty	Pain relief Correction of malalignment and improved mobility
Ankle	Pain, impaired walking	Arthrodesis, ankle replacement (recently)	Pain relief
Foot	Pain, malalignment (hallux valgus), loss of stability	Arthrodesis in mid and hindfoot Resection, fusion of forefoot joints-especially 1st MTP and metatarsal head resection of other toes	Pain relief Improved walking distance from stable foot

Special considerations in RA surgery:

   i. Involvement of multiple joints, disuse atrophy of muscles, tendons and ligaments

  ii. Timing of surgery, when disease is in remission and too late in burnt out disease.

iii. Order of surgery—lower limb joints should be operated first as it may require use of crutches putting strain on upper limb joints. In hand surgery, a proximal to distal direction is followed.

iv. Prosthetic joint replacement may require additional bone graft or augmentation of bone due to poor bone stock.

v. General anesthesia can be difficult in cervical spine involvement

2. **Juvenile idiopathic arthritis:** The complexity of surgeries in children is compounded by the complex deformities, potential for bone growth, emotional maturity of patients and prolonged recovery and rehabilitation. The key component is extensive preoperative planning and appropriate timing.

i. Avoiding loss of ambulation and retaining hand function take priority. The wrist is corrected before MCPs or fingers. In the lower limbs. A painless stable foot is necessary before knee or hip surgeries and hip surgery is done first.

ii. In case of bilateral involvement, both sides are corrected in the same sitting.

iii. Custom made implants may have to be devised due to small bone size.

Procedure	Indication	Outcome
Synovectomy: Reduces volume of inflammatory tissue arthroscopic approach preferred, usually done in knee, hip and wrist	Joint not responding to adequate DMARD, intra-articular steroids	Relieves pain and improves range of movement (ROM)
Surgical soft tissue release	Reduce severe functional impairment combined with joint replacements	Improves ROM
Epiphysiodesis (temporary epiphyseal stapling) Osteotomy	Knee/ankle valgus and limb length discrepancy-before closure of growth plate After growth plate closure	Corrects up to 30 mm of length and 5–20 degree valgus
Total hip arthroplasty (THA) Total knee arthroplasty(TKA)	Painful damaged joints with restricted ROM	Reduces pain and improves function

Female children with positive ANA with high rates of uveitis may require ophthalmic surgery for cataract or glaucoma.

3. **Systemic lupus erythematosus:** Surgeries commonly done are THA, TKA in arthritis, and core decompression of head of femur in early avascular necrosis of head. Surgical emergencies like intestinal obstruction, gangrene or perforation in mesenteric lupus necessitate laparotomy and intestinal resection.

4. **Vascular surgery:** Endovascular stenting or bypass grafting is done for significant stenotic lesions in Takayasu arteritis, aneurysms in Behcets disease and occlusive thrombotic lesions in antiphospholipid syndrome. These are done after controlling disease activity with optimal medical management.

Perioperative management of immunosuppression: This is a fine balance between planning surgery in inactive state of disease to prevent flare while reducing IS agents to avoid perioperative infection. According to ACR/AAHKS guidelines, DMARDs (methotrexate, leflunomide, hydroxychloroquine, sulfasalazine, and/or apremilast) are continued perioperatively, biologics are stopped and surgery done the week following when next dose is due (after 1 dosing cycle), targetted synthetic DMARDs (tofacitinib) stopped 3 days prior, and routine dose of steroid continued rather than giving a supraphysiological stress dose. In severe SLE, mycophenolate mofetil, azathioprine, cyclosporine, tacrolimus, anifrolumab, and voclosporin are continued through surgery, but withheld a week before in mild disease. The medicines are generally restarted 14 days later, after ensuring wound healing and absence of infection.

Conclusion

There is a role for properly timed and planned surgery in arthritis for relief from pain and deformities and improved quality of life. Surgical procedures are life-saving in emergencies in lupus and in salvaging circulation in vasculitis. An adequate peri-operative dialogue with rheumatologist to optimise therapy and reduce infections is necessary.

FURTHER READING

1. Surgical Intervention for Rheumatoid Arthritis and Complication Risks. Marcus Lee, David George, Suan Khor, Michael Elvey and Abbas Rashid University College Hospital, London, United Kingdom.

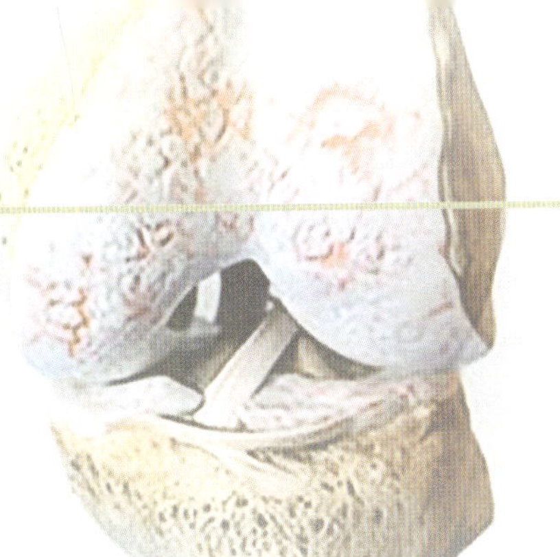

Section

IX

Musculoskeletal Manifestations in Infectious Diseases

Musculoskeletal Manifestations in Tuberculosis

Kavitha Mohanasundaram

INTRODUCTION

Tuberculosis is an endemic disease caused by *Mycobacterium tuberculosis*. Though it is a pulmonary disease dominantly, it can present with a wide array of extrapulmonary manifestations. Musculoskeletal manifestations of tuberculosis need to be identified and treated early for the reduction in morbidity and mortality. With the increasing usage of biologics and Janus kinase inhibitors (JAKi) like tofacitinib, the increase in tuberculosis and its atypical presentations do increase proportionately. This chapter deals with common musculoskeletal manifestations of tuberculosis, its diagnosis and treatment.

Clinical Manifestations

Musculoskeletal manifestations form the third most common extrapulmonary manifestation of tuberculosis next to pleura and lymph nodes. In most cases, this will be the first presentation of tuberculosis in the affected individual. Musculoskeletal manifestations of tuberculosis can be due to direct infection or hematogenous spread of *Mycobacterium tuberculosis* in the joints and tendon or it could be an immunological expression towards the protein. Drugs started to treat tuberculosis have a potential to cause rheumatological illness, like isoniazid induced lupus or pyrazinamide induced hyperuricemia, which may rarely cause gout (Table 57.1).

Table 57.1: Musculoskeletal manifestations of tuberculosis		
Direct Involvement of Joints/spine/soft tissue	*Immunological Reaction*	*Drug Induced*
Tenosynovitis	Poncets disease	Isoniazid–drug Induced Lupus—dominantly arthralgia
TB spine	Erythema nodosum	Pyrazinamide—hyperuricemia
Myositis	Erythema induratum	Quinolones—tendinopathy
Osteomyelitis		
Septic arthritis		
Bursitis/abscess		
Dactylitis		

Direct Involvement

Among the direct manifestations, spondylitis or the Pott's spine is the most common manifestation. The hematogenous spread of tuberculosis bacteria results in granuloma formation, caseous necrosis and eventually destruction of joints unless treated. Thoracic and lumbar vertebrae are commonly affected segments by tuberculosis. Apart from spine, TB involves large joints like hip and knee. TB sacroilitis needs to be suspected in patients with significant low backache with unilateral sacroilitis that crosses the boundaries of joints and involves soft tissue nearby as identified by MRI, HLA-B27 negativity and poor response to conventional treatment for spondyloarthritis. Another joint that is typically involved in tuberculosis is the sternoclavicular joint. A sternoclavicular joint abscess or arthritis needs to be evaluated for tuberculosis particularly when it is an isolated presentation. Dactylitis, bursitis or septic arthritis are other uncommon presentations of a tuberculosis infection.

Immunological Reaction

Poncet's Disease

Poncet's disease is a form of reactive arthritis where the joints are inflamed in a patient with active tuberculosis elsewhere. Unlike Pott's spine, it is not due to direct invasion and *Mycobacterium tuberculosis* cannot be cultured from the joint affected in Poncet's disease. It is considered as a hypersensitive immunological reaction towards tuberculin protein. It is non-destructive, symmetrical poly/pauci articular arthritis affecting large joints—knees, ankle and wrist; knee being the most common joint involved. Complete resolution of arthritis weeks after anti-tubercular therapy is initiated is the norm. Symptomatic treatment with NSAIDs or steroids can sometimes be necessary.

Erythema Nodosum

Erythema nodosum (EN) is a form of panniculitis resulting from inflammation of adipose tissue. Tender, shiny erythematous nodules in the shin of tibia characterize it. The cause of erythema nodosum is often idiopathic; other causes are streptococcal infections, sarcoidosis and tuberculosis. Many times, erythema nodosum is associated with arthritis and a strong Mantoux positivity. EN is associated with constitutional symptoms like fever, malaise and weight loss. It can also be a part of Poncet's disease. It is an example of delayed type IV hypersensitivity reaction. EN as a part of tuberculosis occurs in females aged 20 to 40 years. EN is a predictor for extrapulmonary tuberculosis. Treatment is with anti-tuberculosis therapy according to a country-based regimen.

Drug Induced

The common musculoskeletal symptoms following anti-tubercular therapy are myalgia and arthralgia. Isoniazid (INH) can lead to drug induced lupus (DIL). It is characterized by dominant arthritis, serositis, homogenous ANA positivity (anti-histone antibodies) which improves with stoppage of drug and a short course of steroids. The most important feature is to recognize it early. DIL is an idiosyncratic reaction to isoniazid, where drug exposure leads to lupus-like features. It can start weeks to months after starting INH; it does not involve kidneys or central nervous system and it is usually a milder form of the disease. Pyrazinamide and ethambutol can cause an increase in serum uric acid levels by decreasing renal excretion of uric acid. Pyrazinamide is a strong urate retention agent. Close to 43–100% patients on pyrazinamide show hyperuricemia but acute gouty attack is uncommon. In case of gout attacks, it is managed as per protocols with colchicine, NSAIDs, or short course of steroids. Asymptomatic hyperuricemia does not warrant change of pyrazinamide based regimen. The modified ATT regimen that includes quinolones can lead to tendinopathies.

Conclusion

Musculoskeletal manifestations of tuberculosis, though rare in presentation, are not that uncommon. It should always be kept as a differential diagnosis in endemic regions. With an increase in usage of strong immunosuppression, in all patients with unexplained fever and musculoskeletal manifestations tuberculosis needs to be suspected and actively pursued for. Most patients could be treated with conventional anti-tuberculosis therapy.

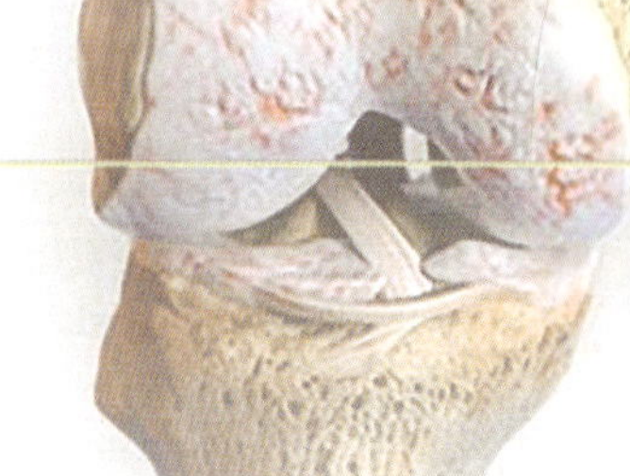

Musculoskeletal Manifestations of Leprosy

Silas Supragya Nelson

INTRODUCTION

Leprosy (Hansen's disease), is an infectious disease caused by *Mycobacterium leprae* (*M. leprae*) and *Mycobacterium lepromatosis* (*M. lepromatosis*) that typically affects the skin and peripheral nervous system, but involvement of upper respiratory tract and eyes is also common.

Incubation period ranges from 2 to 20 years, with an average of 5 years. Transmission, occurs by skin-to-skin contact, nasal secretions or aerosols.

The Ridley-Jopling classification divides leprosy into 5 categories according to the immunological response and number of bacilli in skin lesions, with a spectrum ranging from tuberculoid to lepromatous. The World Health Organization (WHO) classifies patients by the number of skin lesions and the presence of bacilli in skin smear, into paucibacillary (1 to 5 skin lesions, bacteriological index below 2 at all sites) or multibacillary (more than 5 skin lesions; bacteriological index of at least 2 at 1 or more sites).

The rheumatic complaints can vary from mild arthralgia to arthritis mimicking systemic rheumatic diseases.

Epidemiology

Prevalence is inconstant between studies, ranging between 1 and 78%. Rheumatological manifestations occur in 75% of patients with all types of leprosy but are more common in the lepromatous variety. Worldwide India, Brazil and Indonesia, account for 80% of the cases.

Pathophysiology

The proposed mechanisms of pathogenesis include reactional states (Types I and II reaction), inflammation by immune complex deposition and direct infiltration of the synovium by *M. leprae*. Destructive arthropathy by peripheral nerve involvement is also seen (Charcot's disease).

Clinical Features

The arthritis of lepra reactions is acute, symmetrical inflammatory polyarthritis or oligoarthritis affecting small joints of the hands and feet, thus mimicking classic rheumatoid arthritis (RA).

Chronic arthritis is also known to occur in leprosy. It is insidious in onset with periods of exacerbations and remissions involving wrists, knees, MTP joints, MCP and PIP joints of hands.

A high incidence of sacroiliitis (seen in 64%) with erosions was seen, in a cohort of leprosy patients after their leprosy was cured.

Neuropathic arthropathy, also known as Charcot's joints, is characterized by destructive joint involvement with dislocations, pathological fractures and deformities usually involving the weight-bearing joints of the lower limbs, like ankles and the knees. It can be seen in 10% of leprosy.

Swollen hand and feet syndrome (SHFS) first described in 1980 mimics remitting seronegative symmetrical synovitis with pitting edema (RS3PE). The swelling extends from the mid-forearm to MCP joints distally and is pitting. There is inflammation beyond the synovium into the subcutaneous tissue, unlike RA.

Tenosynovitis with arthritis or in isolation can be a presenting feature. Calcaneal enthesopathy and enthesitis are also reported.

Differential Diagnosis

The musculoskeletal manifestations of leprosy mimic various rheumatic diseases and it can pose a diagnostic challenge. Arthritis with tenosynovitis, dactylitis or oligoarthritis of lower limbs can be misdiagnosed as spondyloarthritis. Chronic symmetric arthritis mimics RA and SHFS mimics RS3PE. Ankle arthritis with erythema nodosum can be mistaken for sarcoidosis whereas arthritis with saddle nose and auricular chondritis mimics relapsing polychondritis. Lucio phenomenon can mimic systemic vasculitides.

A combination of arthritis, tenosynovitis with or without paraesthesia or thickened nerves is highly suggestive of leprosy.

Diagnosis

A careful examination for skin lesions (hypoanesthetic macules or patches or erythematous macules, nodules), history of paresthesia, thickened and tender peripheral nerves and sensory and motor neuropathy would clinch the diagnosis in a patient with unexplained rheumatological symptoms, especially if belonging to an endemic area.

The bacilli are not often found in the SF or synovial biopsy specimen, and the diagnosis is clinical. The detection of antibodies to the *M. leprae*-specific phosphoglycolipid-1 along with the PCR is often useful.

Laboratory Features

Inflammatory markers like ESR and CRP are modestly elevated. In one-third of patients, RF, LE cell, and ANAs can be positive, with higher frequency in lepromatous disease. However, anti-CCP antibodies are negative in leprosy or positive in low titres. Anti-neutrophil cytoplasmic antibodies can be positive on immunofluorescence.

Radiology

Radiological abnormalities can range from joint subluxations, dislocations, complete destruction of joints, juxta-articular erosions, periosteitis, bone resorption of terminal phalanges, sacroiliitis and paranasal sinus changes.

Management

The first-line drugs against leprosy are rifampicin, clofazimine and dapsone. According to the WHO, all patients should receive multidrug therapy (MDT). For paucibacillary disease, rifampicin 600 mg monthly single dose and dapsone 100 mg daily for 6 months. For multibacillary disease, rifampicin 600 mg and clofazimine 300 mg monthly along with clofazimine 50 mg and dapsone 100 mg daily for 24 months.

In lepra reactions associated with arthritis, steroids along with MDT are given. Prednisolone is started at a dose of 1 mg/kg/day and gradually tapered by 5 mg every 2–4 weeks. Depending upon the clinical response steroids are given between 4 and 6 months. For severe Type II reactions like erythema nodosum leprosum, MDT and prednisolone are ineffective and other drugs such as clofazimine (300 mg/day) or thalidomide (400 mg/day) are given. TNF-α blocker therapy has proved to be effective in Type II reactions.

Conclusion

Musculoskeletal manifestations of leprosy are common. In endemic countries leprosy should be included in the differential of patients with rheumatic complaints as in the absence of classical cutaneous and peripheral nerve involvement, the rheumatic presentations of leprosy can mimic various rheumatological disorders.

Keywords: Musculoskeletal, leprosy, arthritis.

FURTHER READING

1. Chauhan S, Wakhlu A, Agarwal V. Arthritis in leprosy. *Rheumatology (Oxford)* 2010;49(12):2237–2242. doi: 10.1093/rheumatology/keq264.
2. Schreuder PA, Noto S, Richardus JH. Epidemiologic trends of leprosy for the 21st century. *Clin Dermatol.* 2016;34(1):24–31. doi: 10.1016/j.clindermatol.2015.11.001.
3. World Health O. WHO Expert Committee on Leprosy. World Health Organ Tech Rep Ser. 2012968):1–61, 1 p following 61.
4. El-Gendy H, El-Gohary RM, Shohdy KS, Ragab G. Leprosy masquerading as systemic rheumatic diseases. *J Clin Rheumatol.* 2016;22(5):264–271. doi: 10.1097/RHU.0000000000000379.
5. Rodrigues LC, Lockwood DNJ. Leprosy now: epidemiology, progress, challenges and research gaps. Lancet Infect Dis, 2011;11:464–70.
6. Cossermelli-Messina W, Festa Neto C, Cossermelli W. Articular inflammatory manifestations in patients with different forms of leprosy, *J Rheumatol*, 1998, vol. 25.
7. Albert DA, Weisman MH, Kaplan R. The rheumatic manifestatons of leprosy (Hansen disease). Medicine. 1980;59;442–8.

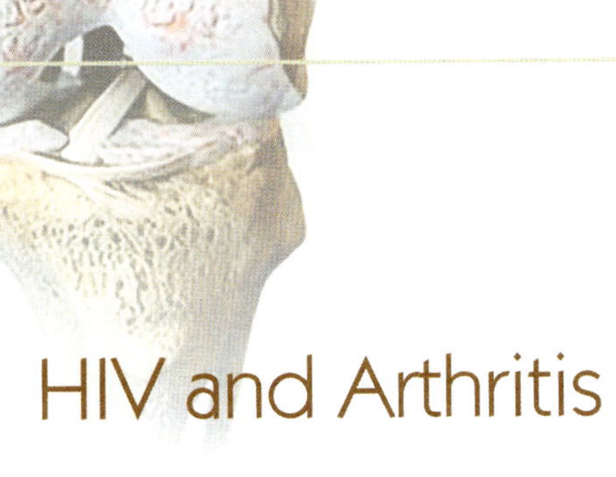

HIV and Arthritis

M Harish Kumar

HIV infection, since its initial description on 1981 has been progressively slowing down globally with patients living longer due to anti-retroviral therapy (ART) and reduced infection incidence. Direct and indirect rheumatic manifestations of the disease depend on the CD4$^+$ count (at count <300 cells/μL. The prevalence before ART varied between 3–70% that reduced to 1.82% post ART. A few serological abnormalities of high anti-CCP titres, RF titres, cryoglobulins, hypergammaglobulins reduce after ART.

This topic will outline the limit itself to the arthritis associated with HIV infection and the manifestations can be classified as follows:

Table 59.1: Musculoskeletal manifestations of arthritis associated with HIV infection	
Arthritis associated with HIV infection	
Unique to HIV infection	a. HIV associated arthralgia (26.67%) b. HIV associated arthritis (2.67%) c. Painful articular syndrome (3.3%)
Manifestation seen in HIV infection	d. Reactive arthritis in HIV (2.3%, 2.67%) e. Psoriatic arthritis (1.67%) f. Undifferentiated spondyloarthritis (8%) g. Hypertrophic pulmonary osteoarthropathy (0.7%)

a. **HIV associated arthralgia:** Arthralgias and myalgias can form a part of early seroconversion syndrome. Up to 26% patients may have unexplained arthralgias. It can be due to circulating viral or host immune complexes and may involve cytokines or bone ischemia. The treatment is symptomatic and non-narcotic analgesia.

b. **HIV associated arthritis:** This is seronegative oligoarthritis that is self-limited lasting less than 6 weeks with no association with HLA B 27 or any other genetic factors and can be seen in up to 12% patients. The common joints involved are the knees (84%), ankles (59%), metatarsophalangeal joints (23%), wrists (41%), elbows (29%), interphalangeal joints (25%) like other viral illness. Synovial fluid is generally sterile. Radiographs can be normal and treatment includes NSAIDs and, in more severe cases, low-dose glucocorticoids. Hydroxychloroquine and sulfasalazine also have been used. Septic arthritis is very rare and was seen in patients with HIV infection due to IV drug abuse. Direct viral replication and growth was not demonstrated from the synovial fluid though the WBC count ranged between 2000–10,000/μL.

c. **Painful articular syndrome:** This is a self-limited syndrome lasting less than 24 hours, with little objective clinical findings characterized by severe bone and joint pain involving the knees predominantly with occasional involvement of elbows and shoulders. This occurs predominantly in the late stages of HIV infection. Aetiology is unknown, and no evidence of synovitis has been found in these patients. Treatment is symptomatic.

d. **Reactive arthritis in HIV:** The incidence of reactive arthritis varies between 2–3% probably due to higher sexually active nature of the population studied and manifested as polyarticular, lower limb-predominant, and progressive; mucocutaneous manifestations like keratoderma blenorrhagicum(14.3%); circinate balanitis and stomatitis occurred in and 9.5% patients. 58% had persistent disease had erosions of foot and/or hand joints and showed early radiological spine or sacroiliac joint changes. Anterior uveitis occurred in 33% of patients. Extensive psoriasiform skin rashes can occur. The clinical overlap makes it difficult sometimes to distinguish HIV-associated reactive arthritis from psoriatic arthritis. HLA-B27 is found in 80 to 90% of patients with HIV-associated reactive arthritis and this association is associated with slower progression to AIDS. NSAIDs are the mainstay of treatment and Indomethacin is recommended, not only for its efficacy, but also for its inhibition of HIV replication that has been observed *in vitro*, which seems to be unique to this NSAID.[7]

e. **Psoriatic arthritis:** The extent of skin involvement with psoriasis can be extensive in HIV+ patients, especially in patients not on anti-retroviral treatment. Cutaneous T cell lymphoma can resemble psoriasis and should be considered in the differential diagnosis of psoriasis in HIV+ individuals. The arthritis in HIV-associated psoriatic arthritis is predominantly polyarticular, lower limb, and progressive while the skin involvement is extensive guttate-plaque admixture and, in contrast to the articular disease, was nonremittive with the onset of AIDS. Anti-retroviral treatment is effective in treating HIV-associated psoriasis and its associated arthritis. Phototherapy may improve the skin rash but also may enhance viral replication, worsen HIV disease, and increase the risk of skin cancer.

f. **Undifferentiated spondyloarthritis:** The incidence of spondyloarthritis in HIV positive patients is less than that of the general population so is the progression to ankylosing spondylitis in patients who had inflammatory backpain and HLAB27 positivity.

g. **Hypertrophic pulmonary osteoarthropathy:** Hypertrophic pulmonary osteoarthropathy affects bones, joints, and soft tissues and can develop in HIV-infected patients with *Pneumocystis jiroveci* pneumonia. It is characterized by severe pain in the lower extremity, digital clubbing, arthralgia, nonpitting edema and periarticular soft tissue involvement of the ankles, knees, and elbows. Radiography reveals extensive periosteal reaction and subperiosteal proliferative changes in the long bones of the lower extremity. A bone scan shows increased uptake along the cortical surfaces. Treatment of *P. jiroveci* pneumonia usually alleviates this condition.

FURTHER READING

1. Fox C, Walker-Bone K. Evolving spectrum of HIV-associated rheumatic syndromes. Best Pract Res Clin Rheumatol. 2015 Apr 1;29(2):244–58.

2. Tehranzadeh J, Ter-Oganesyan RR, Steinbach LS. Musculoskeletal disorders associated with HIV infection and AIDS. Part II: non-infectious musculoskeletal conditions. Skeletal Radiol [Internet]. 2004 Jun [cited 2024 Aug 25];33(6):311–20. Available from: https://pubmed.ncbi.nlm.nih.gov/15127244/

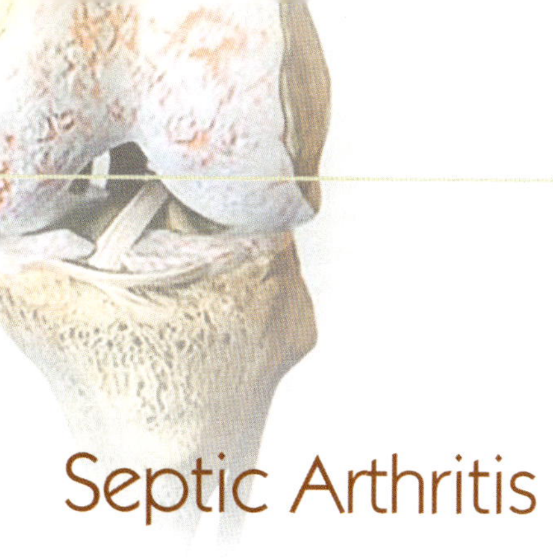

Septic Arthritis

Sowmya Kotha

INTRODUCTION

Septic arthritis, also called infectious arthritis, is a serious condition characterized by an infection in a joint that results in inflammation. As a medical emergency, it necessitates swift diagnosis and treatment to avert joint damage and prevent systemic complications. Typically affecting a single joint, septic arthritis most frequently involves the knee, affecting nearly 50% of cases. Other common sites include the hip, shoulder, elbow, and ankle.

Risk Factors

Children/age >80 years	Intra-articular injections
Diabetes mellitus	Cutaneous infection/ulcers
Rheumatoid arthritis	HIV
Recent joint surgery	Osteoarthritis
Joint prosthesis	Sexual activity/intravenous drug abuse

Septic arthritis occurs when pathogenic microorganisms, most commonly bacteria, invade the synovial fluid and tissues of a joint.

Table 60.1: Pathogenic micro-organisms for septic arthritis in all age groups	
Age Group	*Common Pathogens*
Infants younger than 3 months old	*Staphylococcus aureus* (MSSA and MRSA) Group B streptococci *Klebsiella pneumoniae*
Young children from 3 months to 5 years old	*Staphylococcus aureus* (MSSA and MRSA) Group A *Streptococcus aureus* *Streptococcus pneumoniae*
Children older than 5 years	*Staphylococcus aureus* (MSSA and MRSA) group A Streptococcus.
Adults	*Staphylococcus aureus* (most common), coagulase-negative *Staphylococcus, Streptococcus,* and *Pseudomonas*

The infection typically reaches the joint through three primary routes: hematogenous spread (the most common route), direct inoculation through penetrating trauma or surgical procedures, and contiguous spread from adjacent bone and soft tissue. Once the pathogen enters the joint, it triggers a severe inflammatory response. This response results in the release of inflammatory cytokines and the recruitment of neutrophils, which lead to synovial hyperplasia, joint effusion, and eventual cartilage destruction.

Clinical Features

- Acute onset of joint pain with limitation of movement
- Joint swelling
- Erythema and tenderness
- Fever and malaise
- Sepsis or septic shock

Diagnosis

Diagnosis is typically based on clinical suspicion and is supported by laboratory tests and imaging studies.

1. **Strict aseptic joint aspiration and synovial fluid analysis:** This is the cornerstone of diagnosis. The synovial fluid is analyzed for the following:
   - *Cell count and differential:* A white blood cell count exceeding 50,000 cells/μL and/or neutrophils >90%, along with positive leukocyte esterase (++/+++) and negative glucose, are highly suggestive of septic arthritis. This method has excellent sensitivity and specificity (>90%).
   - *Synovial fluid lactate and calprotectin:* Lactate greater than 10 mg/dl and calprotectin levels above 50 mg/L are supportive of a diagnosis of septic arthritis.
   - *Gram staining and culture:* While Gram staining has limited sensitivity (40 to 70%), cultures are more definitive for identifying pathogens.
   - *Genetic testing:* Polymerase chain reaction (PCR) and metagenomic next-generation sequencing are used to rapidly identify potential pathogenic bacteria.
   - *Crystal analysis:* This test is performed to rule out crystal-induced arthritis.
2. **Blood tests:** Elevated inflammatory markers such as erythrocyte sedimentation rate (ESR) and C-reactive protein (CRP), along with neutrophilic leukocytosis and elevated procalcitonin, are supportive but nonspecific. Blood cultures may also be positive, particularly in cases involving hematogenous spread.
3. **Imaging studies:** Imaging studies can support the diagnosis and assess joint damage. Plain radiographs may reveal soft tissue swelling, widened joint spaces, and, in chronic cases, signs of joint destruction. Ultrasound is useful for detecting effusion, especially in challenging-to-examine joints such as the hip. MRI is the most sensitive modality for identifying early joint and soft tissue changes, as well as the extension of infection into surrounding bone and soft tissue.

Mimics of Septic Arthritis

- Crystal-induced arthropathy
- Reactive arthritis
- Rheumatoid arthritis and other inflammatory arthritis

- Osteomyelitis
- Cellulitis
- Avascular necrosis
- Lyme disease
- Malignancy (metastasis and pigmented villonodular synovitis)
- Transient synovitis

Treatment

Early and appropriate administration of antibiotics, without waiting for bacteriological results, along with immobilization of the affected limb, is essential.

1. **Antibiotic therapy:** Empirical antibiotic therapy should be initiated after synovial fluid aspiration, even before identifying the causative organism. The choice of antibiotic should be guided by the results of the synovial fluid Gram stain or based on clinical suspicion.
   - *Gram-positive coverage:* Since *Staphylococcus aureus* is the most common pathogen, initial therapy typically includes a penicillinase-resistant penicillin (e.g., nafcillin) or a first-generation cephalosporin (e.g., cefazolin). If methicillin-resistant *Staphylococcus aureus* (MRSA) is suspected, vancomycin is the drug of choice.
   - *Gram-negative coverage:* For cases with risk factors for gram-negative infections (e.g., immunosuppression, intravenous drug use), a third-generation cephalosporin (e.g., ceftriaxone) should be used.
   - *Adults with negative Gram stain:* In the absence of specific risk factors for special pathogens or resistant strains, coverage should include *Staphylococcus aureus*, streptococci, and gram-negative bacteria. This can be achieved with cloxacillin plus ceftriaxone or monotherapy with amoxicillin-clavulanate.
   - *Special populations:* For neonates, older adults, and patients with sexually transmitted infections, antibiotics must be tailored to cover specific organisms such as *Neisseria gonorrhoeae* and *Streptococcus agalactiae*.

   Once culture results are available, antibiotic therapy should be adjusted accordingly. The total duration of treatment is typically 3–4 weeks, starting with intravenous antibiotics and transitioning to oral antibiotics as the patient's condition improves. If imaging reveals accompanying osteomyelitis, the treatment duration should be extended to 6 weeks.

2. **Joint drainage:** Effective drainage of the infected synovial fluid is essential for successful treatment. This can be accomplished through the following methods:
   - *Needle aspiration:* Repeated needle aspiration may be adequate for superficial joints, such as the knee.
   - *Arthroscopic drainage:* This minimally invasive technique is preferred for larger joints. Arthroscopic lavage enables direct visualization and thorough cleaning of the joint.
   - *Open surgical drainage:* This approach is necessary when needle aspiration or arthroscopy is not feasible, particularly for deep joints such as the hip.

3. **Supportive care and rehabilitation:** Pain management, immobilization of the affected joint, and physical therapy are essential components of care. Early mobilization and rehabilitation are crucial for preventing joint stiffness and muscle atrophy.

Prognosis

A large cohort study found that the 90-day mortality rate for septic arthritis is 7%, increasing to 22–69% in patients aged 80 years and older. Despite appropriate treatment, septic arthritis can lead to significant complications, including:

- Joint destruction
- Osteomyelitis
- Chronic pain
- Osteonecrosis
- Leg length discrepancies
- Sepsis

FURTHER READING

1. He M, Arthur Vithran DT, Pan L, et al. An update on recent progress of the epidemiology, etiology, diagnosis, and treatment of acute septic arthritis: a review. Front Cell Infect Microbiol. 2023 May
2. Earwood JS, Walker TR, Sue GJC. Septic Arthritis: Diagnosis and Treatment. Am Fam Physician. 2021 Dec
3. Benito, Natividad and Martínez-Pastor, et al. Executive summary: Guidelines for the diagnosis and treatment of septic arthritis in adults and children, developed by the GEIO (SEIMC), SEIP and SECOT. Enfermedades Infecciosas y Microbiologia Clinica, Vol 42, Issue 4,April 2024.